HOPE AND MORTALITY

Psychodynamic Approaches to AIDS and HIV

HOPE AND MORTALITY

Psychodynamic Approaches to AIDS and HIV

edited by

MARK J. BLECHNER

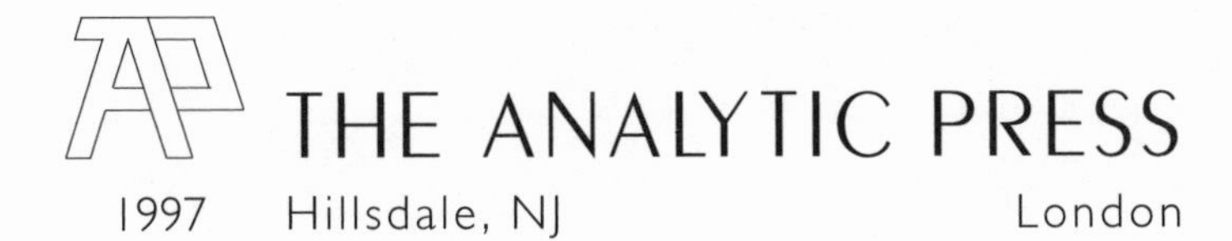
THE ANALYTIC PRESS

1997 Hillsdale, NJ London

Published by
The Analytic Press, Inc.
Editorial Offices:
101 West Street
Hillsdale, New Jersey 07642

Portions of this book appeared previously in M. J. Blechner (1993), Psychoanalysis and HIV disease, *Contemporary Psychoanalysis,* 29:61–80 and M. J. Blechner (1997), Psychological aspects of the AIDS epidemic: A fifteen-year perspective, *Contemporary Psychoanalysis*, 33:89–108.

Library of Congress Cataloging-in-Publication Data

Hope and mortality : psychodynamic approaches to AIDS and HIV / edited by Mark J. Blechner.
p. cm.
Includes bibliographical references and index.
ISBN 0-88163-223-6
1. HIV-positive persons—Mental health. 2. AIDS Disease—Psychological aspects. 3. Psychodynamic psychotherapy I. Blechner, Mark J.
[DNLM: 1. Acquired Immunodeficiency Syndrome— psychology. 2. HIV Infections—psychology. 3. Psychotherapy—methods. 4. Attitude to Death.
WC 503.7 H791 1997]
RC607.A26H664 1997
616.97'92'0019—dc21
DNLM/DLC
for Library of Congress 97-13637
CIP

Printed in the United States of America

10 9 8 7 6 5 4 3 2 1

Dedicated to Hannah and Norbert Blechner

Contents

Contributors xi

Acknowledgments xiii

Introduction xvii

Part 1. PRINCIPLES OF TREATMENT

1. Psychodynamic Approaches to AIDS and HIV 3
Mark J. Blechner

Historical overview 4

AIDS: Course of the illness and medical treatment 11

Psychotherapy with AIDS patients: Goals and countertransference 12

Learning of the HIV-positive diagnosis 14

After the initial diagnosis 17

Timing of interpretations 19

The choice of which issues to work on 21

Psychotherapy with patients in late-stage AIDS 24

Loneliness 25

The role of the psychotherapist 26

The task of the psychotherapist 27

Bereavement 29

Massive bereavement and repeated survivors 31

Survivor guilt 36

Suicidal ideation 37

People having unsafe sex and lying to their partners 38

HIV-related issues in HIV-negative patients 39

HIV testing and AIDS anxiety 42
HIV testing and confidentiality 45
Unconscious factors in assessing one's risk for HIV 46
Cultural determinants in AIDS issues 47
Negotiating safer sex in an unsafe world 48
AIDS and syphilis 52
After the cure 54

2. Modifying Psychotherapeutic Methods When Treating the HIV-Positive Patient **63**
Bertram H. Schaffner

The initial interview: The patient begins life again 65
The therapist's special listening 66
A therapist's dilemma: To touch or not to touch 67
Restoring the patient's autonomy and self-direction 68
Relieving shame: A special challenge 69
The art of probing 70
Unaccustomed roles for the therapist 72
Should the therapist act as moral policeman? 74
Dealing with dementia 75
Death and dying: "Therapist, know thyself" 76

3. Treatment of Children and Parents in Families with AIDS **81**
Seth Aronson

Scope of the problem 82
Issues and themes in grief work with children of parents with AIDS 83
Treatment considerations: Child 87
Treatment considerations: Parent 89
Alternative types of treatment modalities 92
A look to the future 93

4. "Gidget Goes to Sing-Sing": An Interpersonal Therapeutic Approach to HIV-Positive Substance Abusers **97**
Susan Bodnar

Creating an alliance 99
The use of the self 101
Creating chumship 102
Confronting reality issues 103
Integration 104
Adaptations of psychotherapy to a difficult patient population 105
Adaptations to patients with extended life spans 108
Adaptations when someone is close to death 109

Part 2. CASE STUDIES

5. There but for the Grace of . . . : Countertransference During the Psychotherapy of a Young HIV-Positive Woman 115
Sue A. Shapiro

6. Psychotherapy of an AIDS Patient with Dementia 133
Karen Marisak

7. "Playing with Fire": Transference-Countertransference Configurations in the Treatment of a Sexually Compulsive HIV-Positive Gay Man 143
Jean Petrucelli

8. Managing Chronic Loss and Grief: Contrapuntal Needs of an AIDS Patient and His Therapist 163
Richard B. Gartner

9. Disease, Death, and Group Process from a Psychodynamic Point of View 175
Barbara K. Eisold

10. When a Patient Becomes HIV-Positive During Psychotherapy 193
Ernesto Mujica

11. A Heterosexual Male Therapist's Journey of Self-Discovery: Wearing a "Straight"jacket in a Gay Men's Bereavement Group 209
John V. O'Leary

12. Dances with Men: The Impact of Multiple Losses in My Practice of Psychoanalytically Informed Psychotherapy *221*
Susan Bodnar

Index *237*

Contributors

Seth Aronson, Ph.D. is Assistant Director, Child/Adolescent Psychiatry, Jacobi Medical Center and Assistant Professor, Mount Sinai School of Medicine, Yeshiva University and Long Island University.

Mark J. Blechner, Ph.D. (ed.) is Director, HIV Clinical Service, William Alanson White Institute and Clinical Assistant Professor of Psychology, New York University.

Susan Bodnar, Ph.D. is Adjunct Faculty Member, Teacher's College, Columbia University Clinical Psychology Program and in private practice in Manhattan.

Barbara Eisold, Ph.D. is Clinical Supervisor, Yeshiva University and New York University and in private practice in Manhattan.

Richard B. Gartner, Ph.D. is Director, Center for the Study of Psychological Trauma and Founder and Director, Sexual Abuse Program, William Alanson White Institute.

Karen Marisak, Ph.D. is Chief Psychologist, New York Flushing Hospital Medical Center and Adjunct Assistant Professor, Ferkauf Graduate School of Psychology of Yeshiva University.

Ernesto Mujica, Ph.D. is Instructor in Clinical Psychology, Columbia Presbyterian Hospital and Adjunct Assistant Professor, Teacher's College, Columbia University.

John V. O'Leary, Ph.D. is Adjunct Associate Professor, Teacher's College, Columbia University Clinical Psychology Doctoral Program and Supervisor and Teacher, William Alanson White Institute.

Jean Petrucelli, Ph.D. is Codirector, Eating Disorders and Substance Abuse Service, William Alanson White Institute and Supervisor of Psychotherapy, Metropolitan Center for Mental Health in Manhattan.

Bertram H. Schaffner, M.D. is Supervising Analyst and Faculty Member, William Alanson White Institute and Medical Director, HIV Clinical Service, William Alanson White Institute.

Sue A. Shapiro, Ph.D. is Supervising Analyst, New York University Postdoctoral Program in Psychoanalysis and Adjunct Clinical Instructor of Psychiatry, New York University Medical School.

what is
a psychoanalyst
—
someone diff than
maybe also
not a point of view — perspective

Acknowledgments

This book is the product of a true collaboration between individual psychiatrists, psychologists, social workers, internists, institutions, administrators, support staff, friends, and family. It reflects a psychodynamic approach to the psychological effects of AIDS and HIV on individuals, groups, and society as a whole—a point of view that developed first among individual practitioners working in loose association, and which then developed into the HIV Clinical Service of the William Alanson White Institute of Psychiatry, Psychoanalysis, and Psychology in New York City.

I owe thanks to many people who have supported our work. When Dr. Marylou Lionells became director of the William Alanson White Institute, she brought a breath of fresh air and a new vision that opened the way for the development of the HIV Clinical Service. Her foresight and bravery made it all possible, and we are deeply grateful to her. The Board of Directors of the Institute, led by Dr. Charles Harrington, also gave essential support to our work.

I cannot give enough thanks to Dr. Bertram Schaffner, teacher, mentor, colleague, and friend. Dr. Schaffner, an extraordinary humanitarian, is the medical director of the White Institute's HIV Clinical Service. He has been at the forefront of psychiatric efforts to deal with AIDS since the beginning of the epidemic, and he never fails to inspire us with his determination and clinical expertise.

The HIV Clinical Service could not have thrived without the generous efforts of many people. Drs. Margit Winckler, Karen Marisak, and Joyce Barber, as Directors of Referral, have made sure that patients were carefully matched with therapists. Madeline Beusse, fund-raiser and coordinator extraordinaire of the HIV Service, has infused our project with energy, organization, and optimism. Drs. Lyle Tucker and Ernesto Mujica spearheaded our research efforts. Other members of the White Institute community contributed in many valuable ways to our efforts, including Dr. Sondra Wilk, Director of Development, Dr. Clark Sugg, Director of Clinical Services, Dr. Eric Singer, Director of Clinical Education, Ruth Wassell, Chief Psychiatric Social Worker, Diane Amato, Fred Antonoff, Christina Bellamy, Kimberly Fink, Leila Sosa, and José Naranjo.

The Kenworthy-Swift Foundation has given us essential financial support. The Foundation's Director, Dr. Maurice Russell, also contributed his wisdom since our earliest meetings to discuss HIV and mental health.

Dr. Ronald Grossman, a physician who has helped immense numbers of AIDS patients, gave a remarkable lecture to the HIV Service in its earliest days on the medical aspects of AIDS. He has since been a wonderful clinical ally.

Dr. Jack Drescher ably chaired the conference "Psychoanalysis and HIV: Grappling with New Realities" where many of the ideas in this book were first publicly presented. Dr. Mathilde Krim, in her unforgettable keynote address at that conference, inspired many of us to press on, to fight both illness and prejudice.

Dr. Sue Shapiro, a dear friend with whom I share new ideas as they have just taken shape, has inspired me with her candor, open-mindedness, and clinical insights. John Silberman gave me expert legal counsel. Dr. Paul Stepansky and Nancy Liguori of The Analytic Press and Lee Hatfield provided superb editorial advice.

Dr. Jeffrey Blum, a unique friend for 25 years, gave excellent feedback on early drafts of the manuscript. Drs. Richard Gartner, Sandra Buechler, and John O'Leary also read parts of the manuscript, and have contributed to my work in indefinable ways with their warm-hearted generosity and loyal friendship. Jane Bressler, who has impeccably edited nearly everything I have ever written, deserves a lifetime of thanks. Others who have contributed substantially to the growth of my ideas are Dr. Lawrence Mass, Jonathan Ned Katz, and Daniel Kozloff.

Hannah and Norbert Blechner, excellent parents to whom this book is dedicated, have encouraged me throughout my life. The most gratitude belongs to my patients, and those of my colleagues, who have taught us all so much and graced us with their trust.

Introduction

Mark J. Blechner

AIDS has changed all of us, as mental-health professionals, as individual human beings, and as a society. Before the 1980s, none of us thought we would see hundreds of thousands of relatively young people dying of a communicable disease. AIDS has humbled us. Throughout modern Western history, there have been serious sexually transmitted diseases that were incurable. Many of us who came of age in the postpenicillin generation enjoyed a very brief, unusual window in the history of time, a time when it seemed that there were no fatal sexually transmitted diseases, and in which we thought there would be no more. We became arrogant in our faith in modern medicine. AIDS shocked us from our arrogance. It returned the specter of incurable sexually transmitted disease to us, and reminded us that nature is a formidable and clever adversary to human medicine, and will probably always stay one step ahead of man. Through the terrible losses that we have all had to face, AIDS also forced psychological changes in all of us. It forced us to rethink our relation to sickness and health, to mortality, sexuality, drug use, and what we consider valuable in life.

My first patient with AIDS was referred to me in 1982. I was worried about whether I could be of any use to this man. I had no experience working clinically with AIDS patients, but nobody else seemed to know anything more than I did. The referring therapist thought that I, as a gay psychoanalyst in New York, would at least have a greater knowledge base relevant to AIDS than most psychotherapists. In those days, we got our information wherever we could, by word of mouth, from professional journals, and from any other publications. The coverage about AIDS in the mainstream press, like the *New York Times,* was scanty, but I had been following the early medical reports about AIDS, especially the excellent reporting by Dr. Lawrence Mass in the gay publication, the *New York Native*.

I was also fortunate in having an excellent group of colleagues, especially Dr. Bertram Schaffner, with whom I could discuss the special problems that were coming up in working with people with AIDS. Dr. Schaffner, a superb clinician, has been an openly gay psychoanalyst since the 1940s; he is a true pioneer (Schaffner, 1995). When AIDS hit, he was at the center of discussion and leadership. He arranged monthly meetings at his home with other psychotherapists, from all over New York, who were working with AIDS. We discovered that many of us were facing the same problems in our work with AIDS patients. We had all gone through a stage of fearing contagion, which became irrational as we learned more, but was still hard to shed. We had all seen the terrible cost of stigma and shame that added to the pain of having AIDS (Gunther, 1995) and found that we were sometimes stigmatized for working with AIDS patients.

Dr. Schaffner and I also taught a yearly course, AIDS and Psychotherapy, at the White Institute, that was open to all professionals working with AIDS. Each year, the students would express gratitude for the course. Several said that our basic clinical approach was significantly different from that used by most other mental-health providers to people with AIDS. The students certainly appreciated the knowledge they obtained, but what seemed to be most meaningful to them was the chance for intimate personal discussion. Many said that before taking our course they really had had nowhere to discuss the difficult emotions, thoughts, and experiences that they were having when working with HIV, and that this lack was interfering with their clinical effectiveness. At their places of work, which included hospitals, clinics, administrative and policy-making bodies, and other service agencies, it was deemed appropriate to discuss what the patient was going through, but not what the therapist was going through; or, if it was appropriate, the atmosphere was often not safe enough.

So we tried to provide a secure and welcoming atmosphere. We found that when we volunteered our own reactions, some of which had once seemed embarrassing to admit, others would respond, "Yes, I have felt that too, and thought I could never admit that to someone else." Gradually, we came to the realization that working with AIDS brings up the most profound hopes, fears, and anxieties in all of us, the big issues of life and death, hope and despair, how to live, and how to choose.

Robert Browning wrote, in his poem *Andrea del Sarto,* "Ah, but a man's reach should exceed his grasp, or what's a heaven for?" Picking what to reach for, knowing when to let go of an unrealizable goal, setting priorities, finding love—all these are primary issues in life made urgent by the inevitability of death. Most of us try to forget about death most of the time, but working with AIDS patients strips you of that defense. Working with AIDS patients also makes you keenly aware of your individuality. Each person makes these major life choices in very specific ways, and no one knows the right way for anyone else. So working with people with AIDS highlights your own beliefs about how to live, perhaps forcing you to formulate things that you might never have spelled out before, even to yourself.

We were baffled by the denial by much of the population that AIDS was a problem that should concern them. When I first proposed the HIV Clinical Service at the White Institute, some psychoanalysts wondered why we should be involved in such a thing. What could we do for AIDS patients? But too many people were seeing patients with concerns about HIV in their practices and were calling me privately with questions, often with lowered voices. It was as if psychoanalysts were sharing the public shame about AIDS and were ashamed that they had to think about HIV. When I presented a paper about working with AIDS at the White Institute, the problems were made public, and suddenly people asked, "Why aren't we doing something about this?" And thus, thanks in large part to the Institute's new director, Dr. Marylou Lionells, we eventually could set up the HIV Clinical Service at the White Institute.

Orthodox American psychoanalysis has a problematic history with regard to homosexuality (Lewes, 1988), and the stance of many psychoanalysts continues today to reveal the homophobic prejudice of their training (see Isay, 1996; Blechner, 1993, 1994, 1995b, c, d, 1996; Drescher, in press). Orthodox psychoanalysis is also not especially known for addressing the problems of the poor or others who are disadvantaged socially.[1] So it is not surprising that most psychoanalysts were relatively quiet about the AIDS epidemic.

However, the founder of Interpersonal Psychoanalysis, Harry Stack

1. Also, see Altman (1996).

Sullivan, had a different viewpoint and was always concerned with applying psychoanalytic thinking to the most difficult social issues. Sullivan fought prejudice in word and deed. He wrote eloquently about anti-Semitism and what he called anti-Negroism, with startling insights based on self-analysis (Sullivan, 1964). He interviewed black youths in the deep South, one of whom commented: "Dr. Sullivan was one of the nicest white men I'd ever met. It is unusual to have a white man really interested in Negroes. You can't learn to trust white people by one nice one. I guess there are others but I'll bet they're far between" (p. 98).

Sullivan's own homosexuality may have contributed to his being shunned by orthodox psychoanalysis despite his obvious genius. His most famous clinical achievement, the ward for young schizophrenics at the Sheppard and Enoch Pratt Hospital, was also an extraordinary experiment on how the removal of prejudice, homophobic and otherwise, can have a very positive effect on severe psychopathology (Chatelaine, 1981; Blechner, 1992b, 1995a).

It has been gratifying to see so many psychoanalysts, especially young ones, follow Sullivan's example as they take part in the White Institute's HIV Clinical Service. They are eagerly offering their labor, sharing information and insights, and doing really sophisticated, in-depth clinical work with AIDS patients, much of which is described in this book.

The White Institute is a postgraduate training institution, so no one there is really a beginner, but some of our clinicians are 30-something, with perhaps a decade of experience, and some are 80-something, with half a century of experience. They work differently, to be sure, although neither age nor youth has a clear advantage. The ardency, enthusiasm, and energy of relative youth contrasts with the wisdom, patience, and vast knowledge of old age. In this book we present examples of both extremes of experience, and many points in between.

We hope to share with others the depth and flexibility of our work as interpersonal and relational[2] psychoanalysts. In recent years, the AIDS epidemic has become so widespread that every clinician must become well informed about it and the psychological issues it raises. Even those clinicians who do not choose to work with AIDS patients are finding that a patient already in ongoing treatment may become infected with HIV, and other patients may have to deal with rational and irrational fears of infection, the trauma of being tested, and the psychopathological symptomatology related to HIV fears.

My own work for more than fifteen years, as well as the work of my

2. Relational psychoanalysis is an integration of Harry Stack Sullivan's interpersonal psychoanalysis with the best parts of other schools of psychoanalysis.

colleagues in the HIV Clinical Service, has convinced me that modified psychoanalytically oriented treatment can be extremely effective in helping people live with HIV, make the most of the time that they have, confront the difficult challenges when they are sick, and face death with as much dignity and equanimity as possible. I have also found that working with HIV issues brings into question many presumptions of the psychoanalytic theory of psychopathology and clinical action. Working with HIV issues especially challenges many cultural presumptions that are latent in psychoanalytic theory, and it greatly expands the range of effective, yet clearly psychoanalytic, interventions that are clinically possible.

This book is written for all psychiatrists, psychologists, social workers, and other mental-health professionals. Those with extensive knowledge of psychodynamic theory may learn from the book how to apply their knowledge to work with HIV issues and will be challenged to rethink many of their presumptions about psychoanalytic theory and the range of psychological issues that they can treat. Those with experience in HIV and AIDS counseling may find that the book deepens their understanding of the psychodynamics involved in such work and helps them to achieve more meaningful and thoroughgoing change in their patients.

The book begins with several chapters that describe the principles of working with AIDS and HIV. In my chapter, I describe the psychological aspects of the AIDS epidemic and outline the principles of working in psychotherapy both with people with AIDS and people who have concerns about AIDS issues.

Then, Bertram Schaffner, in an especially wise and insightful chapter, describes the changes in psychotherapeutic technique that he has worked out from years of experience working in individual psychotherapy with people with AIDS. He has an admirable sensitivity to issues of self-esteem and hope.

Seth Aronson describes working with children whose parents have AIDS. He focuses on both the parents and the children, in a unique integration of family issues, cultural pressures of the inner city, and individual psychodynamics.

Susan Bodnar describes the experience of working in a hospital setting at St. Clare's, addressing the psychological needs of an inner-city population with AIDS. A modern-day combination of Sullivan, Ferenczi, and Gidget, she highlights the *mutual* accommodation of therapist and patient when they come from very different cultural backgrounds, with an exceptional combination of respect and daring. She teaches her patients about Jewish philosophy, while they teach her, with astonishing directness, about her own vulnerabilities, and they all learn about being "more simply human than otherwise."

These first four chapters cover many of the basic principles of working with AIDS and HIV issues. While they all contain substantial clinical material, the chapters that follow are primarily clinical case reports. They report, in much greater detail, the long-term work with patients in psychodynamic psychotherapy, highlighting a particular clinical difficulty.

Sue Shapiro describes vividly how her own experience of the counterculture in the 1960s and of multiple deaths in her family shapes the way she hears her patient's own countercultural leanings in a different era. She also candidly shares her self-analytic insights as she finds a way between supporting and questioning her patient's exploration of alternative treatments to traditional Western medicine.

Karen Marisak tackles a difficult problem: adjusting her psychotherapeutic approach with a patient whose mental functioning gradually deteriorates from AIDS dementia. One cannot help being impressed by her patience and her attention to the constructive and hope-sustaining value of fantasy, even when it is completely unrealistic.

How do you work psychotherapeutically with someone who is sexually compulsive? Jean Petrucelli finds a way to develop symbolic intimacy with a gay man whose history of sexual abuse has led to a dissociation of feeling and sexuality. Her account has a marvelous poignancy and playfulness as she thinks theory, and he responds in the most basic, visceral way to her physical and emotional presence.

Richard Gartner, in working with a gay man with AIDS, learns about the effects of having all of your friends and romantic partners die. He observes the numbing effects of multiple loss on his patient and himself, and shows us how important it is to analyze our own unique attitudes toward death.

Barbara Eisold presents a very personal account of leading a support group for gay men with AIDS. She eschews standard models of group treatment as she explores the benefits and pitfalls of a very individualized attention within a group format. She also learns a lot about herself, recovering her own near-death memories.

Ernesto Mujica tells the painful tale of a patient who becomes HIV-positive in the course of his psychotherapy. His account raises important questions about the individual responsibility of patient and therapist, and pays close attention to processes of denial and dissociation about issues of HIV risk.

John O'Leary's chapter is, as far as I know, unique in the psychological literature related to sexual orientation. O'Leary finds himself in an uncomfortable situation, a *heterosexual closet*, as he runs a therapy group for HIV-negative gay men who have lost someone to AIDS. As he struggles to "come out of the closet," he comes to understand fear of exposure, secrecy, prejudice, homophobia, and the relationship of politics and psychological experience. His candid discovery of prejudice is in the tradition of trailblazing works such as Griffin's *Black Like Me*.

In good psychotherapy, not only the patient is changed. The therapist who uses all of her psychic resources inevitably is also changed. Susan Bodnar, in her second chapter, "Dances with Men," shows how her extensive work at Roosevelt Hospital with people with AIDS—mostly gay, bisexual, and transgendered—led to her working through her own untimely loss of her husband and to her finding a way to move forward in her life.

Principles of Interpersonal Psychoanalysis

All of the casework described in this book is influenced by the principles of interpersonal and relational psychoanalysis. In the briefest manner, I will outline here the fundamental principles of this kind of psychotherapeutic work.

1. The patient has a right to set the goals of his treatment.
2. The psychotherapist should consider how the symptomatology helps the patient adapt to life, not only how it is dysfunctional. To do this effectively, the psychotherapist must have a detailed knowledge of the patient's current and past life. The analysis of unconscious experience, through dreams and other aspects of the patient's communications, helps clarify the dynamics of the patient's way of living.
3. The therapeutic action of psychoanalysis is facilitated by the relationship with the therapist. This relationship helps identify persistent patterns in living and experiencing other people, which the therapist can outline, making possible insight and change. The relationship also helps the patient in and of itself, because it may make up for deficits in the patient's development.
4. Analysis of transference and countertransference are essential aspects of the therapeutic work and are best achieved through a collaborative exploration between patient and therapist. This means examining the personal emotions and perceptions evoked in both the patient and therapist by one another. Analysis of these interactions allows clarification of the enduring personality patterns of the patient, which then makes change possible. The therapist's countertransference must also be taken into account. The special characteristics, personality traits, and cul-

> tural background of the therapist must be factored into an understanding of the patient's reactions.

Of course, interpersonal and relational psychoanalytic theory is much more complex than this. Readers interested in greater detail may wish to consult some basic reference works, such as Sullivan (1953), Fromm-Reichmann (1950), Mitchell (1988), and Lionells et al. (1995).

I believe, however, that the case examples presented here teach by illustration. Though the therapists all share certain theoretical principles, they are as different and unique as their patients. They differ in race, ethnicity, sexual orientation, marital status, religious and cultural backgrounds, and in much more precise, unclassifiable ways that are nevertheless communicated in the details, style, and tone of their reports. The therapists grew up in different eras, in different socioeconomic conditions, and have varying amounts of experience (they range in age from 34 to 84). These factors must be taken into account in considering one's therapeutic impact.

All of the therapies described in this book are full of life, revealing the give-and-take of two individual presences. In editing the book, I have avoided tampering with the individual voices of the therapists. I want the reader to have a vivid, first-hand experience of what the therapists are like in the consulting room—how they speak, work, and think. Psychoanalytic and psychodynamic treatments are nothing if they are not alive, *dynamic* in both senses of the word (addressing psychic forces and lively). The aim of this book is to teach about AIDS issues and to show, as well, how modern thinking in psychoanalysis is put into practice.

References

Altman, N. (1995), *The Analyst in the Inner City*. Hillsdale, NJ: The Analytic Press.

Blechner, M. J. (1992), Psychoanalysis, homophobia, racism, and anti-Semitism: Introduction. Presented at the conference of the William Alanson White Society, "The Experience of Hating and Being Hated," November 18, New York.

——— (1993), Homophobia in psychoanalytic writing and practice. *Psychoanal. Dial.*, 3:627–637.

——— (1994), Review of Darlene Ehrenberg's *The Intimate Edge*. *Psychoanal. Dial.*, 4:283–292.

——— (1995a), Schizophrenia. In: *Handbook of Interpersonal Psycho-*

analysis, ed. M. Lionells, J. Fiscalini, C. Mann & D. B. Stern. Hillsdale, NJ: The Analytic Press, pp. 375–396.

——— (1995b), The shaping of psychoanalytic theory and practice by cultural and personal biases about sexuality. In: *Disorienting Sexuality,* ed. T. Domenici & R. Lesser. New York: Routledge, pp. 265–288.

——— (1995c), The interaction of societal prejudice with psychodiagnosis and treatment aims. *Round Robin,* September, pp. 10–14.

——— (1995d), Homosexuality, homophobia, and clinical psychoanalysis. Presented to the Graduate Faculty, New School for Social Research, March 9.

——— (1996), Psychoanalysis in and out of the closet. In: *The Therapist as a Person,* ed. B. Gerson. Hillsdale, NJ: The Analytic Press.

Chatelaine, K. (1981), *Harry Stack Sullivan.* Washington, DC: University Press of America.

Drescher, J. (in press), Changing psychoanalytic attitudes toward homosexuality: From Rosa K to disorienting sexuality. *Gender & Psychoanal.*

Fromm-Reichmann, F. (1950), *Principles of Intensive Psychotherapy.* Chicago: University of Chicago Press.

Gunther, H. C. (1995), The impact of homophobia and other social biases on AIDS. *Public Media Center Report,* pp. 1–38.

Isay, R. (1996), *Becoming Gay.* New York: Pantheon.

Lewes, K. (1988), *The Psychoanalytic Theory of Male Homosexuality.* New York: Simon & Schuster.

Lionells, M., Mann, C., Fiscalini, J. & Stern, D., eds. (1995), *Handbook of Interpersonal Psychoanalysis.* Hillsdale, NJ: The Analytic Press.

Mitchell, S. (1988), *Relational Concepts in Psychoanalysis.* Cambridge: Harvard University Press.

Schaffner, B. (1995), The difficulty of being a gay psychoanalyst during the last 50 years. In: *Disorienting Sexuality,* ed. T. Domenici & R. Lesser. New York: Routledge, pp. 243–254.

Sullivan, H. S. (1953), *The Interpersonal Theory of Psychiatry.* New York: Norton.

——— (1964), *The Fusion of Psychiatry and Social Science.* New York: Norton.

Part 1

PRINCIPLES OF TREATMENT

1 Psychodynamic Approaches to AIDS and HIV

Mark J. Blechner

In this chapter, I address many aspects of AIDS. First, in order to provide a historical perspective, I tell, from my own viewpoint, how the AIDS epidemic evolved and how psychological attitudes, among patients and all of society, have shifted. In particular, I explore ways in which psychoanalysis can help us understand the terrible, irrational reactions that have made the AIDS epidemic not only a medical tragedy, but a psychological tragedy for society and individuals. I then describe what we have learned, from a psychodynamic perspective, about working with people with AIDS and people with concerns about HIV. We have learned many ways in which psychoanalytic principles can be adapted and expanded to allow all psychotherapists, in many difficult situations, to help people with AIDS and those who love them and take care of them.

Psychological Aspects of the AIDS Epidemic: Historical Overview

In the earliest years, AIDS was a mystery. In 1980, the "epidemic," as a recognized entity, did not exist. At that time, however, I personally knew one man, James Allen, who was in his late 20s and was having unusual medical problems. He was first diagnosed with shingles, then with Hodgkin's disease, but his medical progress did not fit the diagnoses. By 1981, we knew the rumors of some horrible disease that was striking mainly gay men, but no one knew how it was caused, whether it was contagious, or much of anything else; we knew only that young men were becoming very sick and were dying rather quickly. James now knew that he had this disease, whatever it was. The last time I saw him was at the opera; he was walking feebly with a cane. He said, "Next year at this time, I will be the late James Allen." He was right. I still remember the shock of seeing a friend, so young and with so much promise, become so debilitated and resigned to death. Now I have seen the same thing happen, over and over, with patients, colleagues, and friends, and the cumulative effect is one of numbing, shock, and despair.

At first, the disease was thought to be restricted to gay men, and was dubbed GRID (Gay-Related Immune Disorder). Colloquially, some people referred to Kaposi's sarcoma as the "gay cancer." In early 1983, I heard a man at a party bragging cheerfully that he had had the gay cancer and was cured of it. He was wrong. This man's bravado was an example of simple reaction formation, a reversal of the terror that was the most common emotion at the time in gay men. No one knew who would next get the illness. No organism had been identified as causative, and no marker had been identified that would predict who was contagious or who would next be stricken. Physicians and psychotherapists alike had no idea whether one could get the illness just by being with the patient.

In this period of mystery and terror, irrational ideas were rampant and caused much havoc. Psychoanalysis is the field that established the irrational and the unconscious as areas worthy of study. So what can we learn from psychoanalysis about the irrational thinking that is aroused by AIDS? Freud and Sullivan have taught us how all aspects of human psychology—memory, perception, thinking, and reasoning—can be altered by intense emotional concerns. To understand HIV and the irrational attitudes connected with it, one ought to invoke two of the great concepts of psychoanalysis—Freud's concept of *wish-fulfillment,* and Sullivan's notion of the *not-me*. Both of these concepts were intended to describe the processes of individual psychology, but both of them can be expanded to describe the group psychological processes of distortion and myth-making that we have seen rampant in the AIDS epidemic and that still continue today.

Freud (1900, 1901) postulated that when we are under great emotional stress, our reasoning can become illogical by the same mechanisms that usually make our dreams so strange. Our waking thoughts can be distorted by primary processes and ego defenses, like displacement, repression, denial, and reaction formation. I think that the great fear and panic invoked by the AIDS epidemic have led to those kinds of distorted thinking. The distortions, however, have not been only on the level of individual psychology, but also on the level of large groups, and ultimately all of society. Over and over during the AIDS epidemic we have seen the distortions of individuals coalescing into distorted group beliefs, which we also call "myths." Because these myths fulfill such a strong psychological need, they are very hard to dispel.

And what are the AIDS myths that have been produced? There have been many; but a common theme of the myths is that the AIDS epidemic affects someone who is "not-me," to use Sullivan's term. In the beginning of the epidemic, when so few facts were available, everyone wanted to project the danger of the epidemic onto someone else, and the most convenient targets were groups that are hated or looked down upon. For instance, in the beginning of the epidemic, there was a rumor among white gay men that the only people getting AIDS were those who were sleeping with black men. Meanwhile, as Washington (1995) has documented, black men thought the opposite, that AIDS was a disease of white gay men and that black men could be safe as long as they only slept with each other. Of course, both groups were wrong. The same phenomenon is repeating today in many parts of the world; in Cambodia, for example, a poll showed that most hospital nurses believe that AIDS is a disease of foreigners, and that it cannot be passed between Cambodians (Shenon, 1996).

In 1983, things changed dramatically. A virus was finally isolated that was presumed to cause AIDS, which was eventually called "HIV" (human immunodeficiency virus). Soon thereafter, there was a blood test for antibodies to the virus. Now there was a name for what was happening and a biological marker for the presumed cause of the illness. It was recognized that the illness was contagious through sexual contact or exchange of blood products, and that those who had already acquired the virus but were asymptomatic could be identified.

The psychological effect of this medical discovery was of tremendous importance. What had previously been blind terror now became more concrete. Those who were ill had some idea of what was going on, although much was still unknown. Those who were HIV-negative could find out, and could react to that news (with relief, guilt, or other reactions). A class of psychopathology, the "worried well," became more precise, now that it could be determined who was well in a biological sense. And in those days, with more concreteness to the horror, there was concomitantly more *hope* as well. Science had developed vaccines against other viral diseases. Surely, people thought, science would find a way to cure or prevent AIDS. People spoke of a cure around the corner, and, on April 23, 1984, Margaret Heckler, secretary of health and human services, even made an official government announcement to that effect. Such events often crossed the border into denial; there was a pervasive belief among white American heterosexuals that the illness was restricted primarily to "risk groups"—gay men, IV drug users, hemophiliacs, and Haitians. This was maintained despite the fact that in Africa it was clear the epidemic, for the most part, was affecting heterosexuals, but this was explained away vaguely as a result of open chancre sores caused by other sexually transmitted diseases, or perhaps by female circumcision or some other exotic practices—anything to prove that the African is "not-me." Denial is a strong defense, and it finds ways to produce all sorts of flimsy data that seem to acquire merit through the wish that they be true. There was a continual attempt to ascribe AIDS to the "other," the "not-me." Gay men in their 20s originally thought that they were safe as long as they avoided sex with people over 30. The subsequent upsurge in HIV infection in young people proved how wrong and tragic such misconceptions are.

"Risk groups," the term used by epidemiologists, was itself very misleading. It implied that those who were not part of the risk groups were not at risk of contracting HIV. Perhaps "highest risk" groups would have been more accurate and allowed for less denial. But the damage has been done, and the epidemic has spread among heterosexuals who were once not included in the risk groups (see Blechner, 1986). In the 1990s, women became the fastest growing group affected by AIDS in the United States; their numbers were increasing by 45 percent each year.[1]

Over time, our understanding of the nature and epidemiology of the disease has changed, and with it our assessment of fears of it. Yesterday's irrationality has more than once become today's reality, and vice versa. In the mid 1980s, when it was thought that only 30 percent of sero-positive individuals would progress to AIDS, the belief that one was facing certain death from HIV infection was considered irrational. Since then, the estimate has been gradually moved upward, so that

1. HIV Center for Clinical and Behavioral Studies Report, New York, New York State Psychiatric Institute, Vol. 1, May 1991.

some clinicians felt that with time, nearly all HIV-infected individuals would contract the disease. This most dire outlook was somewhat tempered when a certain group of individuals, the "nonprogressors," seemed not to become symptomatic despite HIV infection. One reason for nonprogression was clarified in 1996, when it was found that a genetic anomaly produced a natural resistance to the HIV virus in about one person in 100 among Caucasians.

In addition, there is more hope than ever that a medical solution will be found, and that AIDS will shift from being a terminal illness to a chronic, manageable one, like diabetes, or even a totally curable or preventable one. Also, we now know that the human immunodeficiency virus is transmitted only through the transfer of blood products or body fluids directly into the bloodstream or through mucous membranes, and so fears of casual contact are unfounded. There is no danger that a psychotherapist who chooses to work with AIDS patients will get AIDS from them.

But AIDS is psychologically threatening. It is not acceptable to the unconscious. AIDS, somewhat like schizophrenia and the Holocaust, is a horrifying, death-in-life situation that we would like not to exist, so much so that denials are repeatedly propagated in the public consciousness that these things, in fact, do not exist. The Holocaust didn't happen, claim some historians. Schizophrenia is not an illness, claim some psychiatrists. And the so-called general population does not have to worry about AIDS, say some public health officials. Since there can be a latency period of many years between infection with the HIV virus and the onset of symptomatic AIDS, it may be possible to maintain such a myth until it is too late, but already the rising incidence of HIV infection among teenagers is an alarming sign.

Many other myths continue to develop about AIDS, driven by the wish for immunity from the disease. As mentioned above, young gay men in their 20s often think that they are safe from the virus as long as they have sex only with others younger than 30. Also, physicians have studied AIDS primarily in men. Until 1991, the Centers for Disease Control's definition of AIDS did not even mention several opportunistic infections that occur only in women, such as various forms of cancer and pelvic inflammatory disease, so that many women are not properly diagnosed. One physician put it this way: "In the United States, women don't get AIDS; they just die of it." It is important for a psychotherapist to challenge such myths, but he cannot do so unless he has educated himself and overcome his own unconscious tendencies toward such irrational beliefs.

The level of irrationality about AIDS produces the most bizarre belief systems. Think about the following question: What do you believe is the chance that two gay men who are HIV-negative can transmit the HIV virus to one another during anal intercourse? Herek and Capitanio (1993) studied this question. They found that about half of their subjects believed there was a strong chance of HIV transmission between two uninfected homosexual men. Of course, the correct answer is zero. But their study shows how many people irrationally connect HIV transmission with specific behaviors. If anal intercourse is one of the most efficient ways of spreading the HIV virus, then any act of anal intercourse is thought to cause AIDS. This is not so different from the principle of von Domarus (1944) that has been applied to schizophrenic reasoning, in which things that are merely associated with one another are seen to have a causal or inclusive relationship. For example, a schizophrenic may think, "If my mother's name is Mary, and Mary is the mother of God, then I am God." You may think that only schizophrenics think like this, but as Freud and Jung have shown us, when we are under great emotional pressure we are all capable of reasoning like madmen.

One would like to think that after a decade and a half of AIDS, we would see the most severe forms of irrationality, fear, and ignorance disappearing. But we are not. In 1995, a group of gay political leaders were to meet with President Clinton at the White House. Secret Service agents who frisked them wore rubber gloves as a precaution against contracting AIDS. What was their reasoning? The same von Domarus principle seems to have been at work. Many gay people have AIDS. Therefore, all gay people have AIDS. Doctors use rubber gloves when examining AIDS patients where there are bodily fluids. So rubber gloves will prevent me from getting AIDS when frisking gay men. Of course, the fact is that you cannot get AIDS by frisking anyone, with or without gloves. But if such ignorance exists in the American federal government, what can we expect of those with less education and less public responsibility?

Irrational beliefs and prejudice also limit research into issues of drug use and sexuality that are crucial to AIDS transmission. June Osborn (1992), as chair of the National Commission on AIDS, said that "even our most basic efforts to better understand and respond to this new plague have been hampered. Efforts have been made to constrain or forbid behavioral research." Even though we know that clean needles dramatically reduce the spread of HIV among IV drug users (Karel, 1993; Hausman, 1993), most states do not allow ready access to such clean needles, because of a fear that this will encourage drug use. Even though anal intercourse is known to be the most efficient means of transmitting HIV sexually, the government has refused funding for literature that would explicitly mention anal intercourse, for fear that it will encourage such behavior. The unconscious ideas here are that if you talk about a behavior, you encourage it. Not talking or thinking about it causes the behavior to be less present. Both of these ideas are false and dangerous. Needle-exchange programs do not cause more people to be drug addicts, and safe-sex education does not increase the rate of anal intercourse. But while such programs are discouraged in Congress, AIDS has been spreading relentlessly.

The press has shown many of the same psychological defenses and prejudices in its coverage of AIDS news, a combination of denial and dissociation of the not-me. When Legionnaire's disease took 29 lives in 1976, it made instant front-page news, and the government made immediate pronouncements about its medical significance. For the first 30 days of the Legionnaire's epidemic, the *New York Times* included stories on it every day but one, and put the story on the front page 11 times. With AIDS, news coverage was scanty for years in mainstream papers. By the end of 1982, two years into the epidemic, the *New York Times* had printed only six articles about the epidemic, none of them on the front page. When President Reagan first mentioned AIDS in a public address in 1987, more than 20,000 people had already died of the disease (Shilts, 1987, p. 596). The fact that it was mostly gay men and IV drug users who were the first victims of the illness surely was responsible. Yet, over 10,000 hemophiliacs were also infected with HIV, because of reckless behavior of government agencies and corporations that did not adequately test and monitor the blood supply. Such negligence has often been settled legally, but that will not cure the "Committee of 10,000" hemophiliacs with AIDS.

Because of the government's irrationality, many people involved in the AIDS epidemic became political activists. In the 1980s, political activities definitely helped many AIDS patients whom I saw in psychotherapy feel hopeful and supported by the community. To a certain degree, in the 1980s this hope seemed justified. This was the era of the cure being around the corner. Every few months, there was the new great hope, the new magic medicine. There was Suramin, which turned out to be ineffective and extremely toxic. People flew to Paris to get HPA-23, thinking that it was the great cure that was available only to the rich and well-connected. They were wrong; it didn't work. AL-721, a derivative of egg yolks from Israel, was another great hope, and it did not have a high level of toxicity. People began to drink homemade egg-yolk concoctions, which did virtually no harm, but ultimately not much good either. Chinese cucumber, Ribaviran, thermal treatment of the blood, and many other remedies were tried. With each, there was a flurry of great hope, and then, when the results did not hold up, first there was denial, then disappointment.

There was even belief that psychological ministrations would turn the disease around. People like Louise Hay told large groups of patients that AIDS could be healed by positive thinking, and while this led many people to have great hope, it was especially cruel when they became sicker. Then, not only did they have to deal with a worsening medical condition, they also felt that it was a personal and moral failure.[2]

By the early 1990s, there was less anger and less hope. The popular slogan, "Be here for the cure," started to take on a cruel sound; I heard AIDS patients in psychotherapy speaking much less confidently that a cure would be found in their lifetimes. There was still rage, but it became more diffuse, and less clearly directed at any available "enemy." This despair became almost institutionalized at the 1994 International AIDS Conference, when scientists agreed to hold the conference only every two years, instead of annually. This was tantamount to a public acknowledgment of loss of hope by science and government, and the reflection of this public despair onto individual psychology was very debilitating.

Nevertheless, on the positive side, there was a great deal of medical progress, especially in treating and preventing individual opportunistic infections. And we learned how to tell much better where someone is in the progress of the disease, thanks to various markers of the capacity of the immune system and of the viral load (Mellors et al., 1996). These markers allowed more sophisticated medical attacks directly against the HIV virus.

There was a dramatic shift around 1996, when results became public that a new class of drugs, the protease inhibitors, could actually cause the HIV virus to relent. When given with at least two other antivirals, the "cocktail" of medications could cause the HIV virus to be undetectable in the blood. This was the first time that the actual immune

2. Monette (1994) has written eloquently about this experience. "I'd struggled with the various denial systems purveyed by a raft of New Age gurus, the ones who filled whole auditoriums in Hollywood, promising that if we loved ourselves enough we wouldn't die. Tapes available at the door, $29.95, no checks please. Courses in miracles, follow the white light, anger will kill you faster than AIDS. Et cetera.

"The worst. Designed to make people feel that if they *did* get sicker, they weren't loving their lesions enough, or keeping up with their positive imaging. In a word, the dying were losers. I had watched too many acquaintances, gulled into fairyland by Louise and Marianne, turn bitterly away from them when the disease began to win. The New Age ladies drew the line at visiting the dying. Play those tapes, boys, louder and louder. My neighbor Billy, who'd gloried in his role as Ed McMahon on the Wednesday evening "Hayrides," went into a black depression when the lesions swarmed over his face. The New Age stopped returning his calls. He hanged himself from the clothes bar in his closet, undiscovered for three days, till a pair of lesbian friends from back East arrived for the weekend and broke down the door" (p. 83).

deficiency seemed to be significantly *reversed;* it became possible to hope that AIDS would no longer be an inevitable progression toward death, with medications able only to slow the relentless decline. Some people who had been extremely ill and hopeless were now able to function again, as their T-cell counts climbed. Having resigned themselves to death, they suddenly faced the prospect of remission or even recovery.

Unfortunately, there are still many questions about the protease inhibitors. They simply do not work for some patients, variously estimated to be about a third of those in treatment. We do not know if their effect is long-lasting, or whether they will eventually lose their effectiveness as the virus mutates and "outsmarts" them. The side effects of the medications are so severe for some people that they cannot tolerate them. For some people, the apparent improvement in the lab results does not translate into medical improvement. I worked with one man who took the protease inhibitors, and whose viral load was reduced to zero. But he remained ill and weak. He said to me, "They say that on paper I should be recovering, but I'm still in pain and getting sicker and weaker." He died not long after.

So once again we are facing the dialectic between hope and despair, with the outcome still to be determined. The wish for the epidemic to be over is so strong that there are many misleading, exaggerated statements of the current medical facts. People with AIDS are fearing that premature optimism will lead their caretakers, and society in general, to lessen support of them, while they continue to suffer. Also, because the combination therapies are extremely costly, they are not benefiting most of the estimated 28 million people infected with HIV worldwide, of whom the majority are in impoverished countries. There is also the tremendous danger that young people will now be less careful about avoiding HIV transmission, thinking, wrongly, that they can be cured.

AIDS: Course of the Illness and Medical Treatment

AIDS is a horrible illness that gradually debilitates the body's normal immune system. Consequently, the person with AIDS suffers a sequence of varied and unusual illnesses known as "opportunistic infections." These include, most commonly, pneumocystis carinii pneumonia (PCP), various herpes infections, a heretofore rare form of cancer known as Kaposi's sarcoma, cytomegalovirus infection, oral candidiaisis, various lymphomas and parasites; the entire list is quite a bit longer, and new opportunistic infections are continually being discovered.

The medical treatment of AIDS usually proceeds on two tracks. In the first track of treatment, the human immunodeficiency virus (HIV), which is presumed to cause AIDS, is attacked directly, with medications that interfere with the replication of the virus and its destruction of the immune system. The second track is to treat the opportunistic infections individually as they appear, or to try to prevent their appearance by preventive medications. For example, the onset of PCP may be forestalled by Bactrim or other oral medication. The advances in treatment have allowed AIDS patients to live longer than when the syndrome was first identified. In time, the HIV virus, which is presumed to cause the immunodeficiency, also directly attacks the nervous system, leading to various cognitive deficits and dementia. In nearly all cases, the patient's physical condition deteriorates under the onslaught of all these diseases, until death.[3]

AIDS is dreadful in its course and in the multiplicity of its manifestations. In addition, unlike many other epidemics of the past, most of its victims have been in the prime of life, when careers are blossoming and life is usually lived to the fullest. They feel robbed of their maturity. So far, the group with the highest incidence of AIDS in America has been gay men. The second highest incidence has been among intravenous drug users, and this group currently has the highest rate of increase of the disease. The IV drug users are also predominantly black or Hispanic, probably about 80 percent. Other groups that are hard hit are hemophiliacs and the sexual partners of bisexual men and IV drug users, and their newborn children. In Africa, however, these specially victimized groups do not pertain, and it is unknown if and when the distribution of the disease in Western countries will change, although there are clear signs that the frequency of AIDS among heterosexuals who are not drug users is on the rise.

Psychotherapy with AIDS Patients: Goals and Countertransference

With the current medical advances, most people who are HIV-positive can count on living for years, 10 or even more, and that is enough time for a patient with long-standing interpersonal difficulties to make very

3. The new medications have suggested the possibility that death may not be inevitable, but, as I write this, it is too soon to know. Also, it seems that some percentage, perhaps one in 20 people who are HIV-infected, have so far not progressed to AIDS for 10 or more years. Whether they have a less dangerous form of the virus or some other factor is at work is still under study (Cao et al., 1995; Pantaleo et al., 1995). The San

good use of psychotherapy. The question is, how should one conduct psychotherapy with people with AIDS? What modifications are necessary in our work, and also, what does work with AIDS patients teach us about doing better psychotherapy with all patients?

At the William Alanson White Institute, we have been adapting the principles of interpersonal psychoanalysis to working with AIDS. The interpersonal approach to psychopathology is guided by the fundamental question of William Alanson White: "What is the patient trying to do?" (Sullivan, 1924, p. 8). We need to formulate this question with the patient and then determine whether we can and should help him or her to do it, and if so, how (Blechner, 1995a). Psychotherapy of the person with AIDS usually has three basic aims: (1) to help him or her take advantage of life-enhancing medical care; (2) to resolve or come to terms with whatever psychological issues are troubling; and (3) to make the best use of the time that remains.

The therapist of a person with AIDS needs to have two kinds of knowledge: medical and psychological. The therapist needs a good basic knowledge of the facts of AIDS, how the illness progresses, what are the signposts of significant changes, and how the patient's relationship with his internist can be made more or less effective because of psychological factors. The therapist also needs an understanding of human defenses, including the fact that some defenses, like denial, can serve patients well in going on with their lives. And just as important, the therapist needs to have self-knowledge.

In the early days of psychoanalysis, the analyst's own emotional reaction, the countertransference, was thought to be an impediment to effective treatment. Today, we have learned that the countertransference is one of the analyst's most useful tools. By examining your own emotional reactions, no matter how irrational or disturbing, you can learn important things about the psychodynamics of your patient, and those of his family and caregivers. When Dr. Bertram Schaffner and I started to teach psychotherapists who work with AIDS patients, we discovered that the most frequent problem they face is not knowing how to use their countertransference productively and not having a setting where they can safely and openly discuss their emotional reactions. Most therapists do not have trouble when their countertransference emotions are kindly, good feelings. But when working with severely ill and dying patients, the therapist can have uncanny, dreadful, or painful emotions,

---

Francisco City Clinic cohort study (Buchbinder et al., 1993) found that 8 percent of men who were infected between 10 and 15 years ago remain healthy today, with only minor immunologic abnormalities. It is now known that about 1 percent of Caucasians possess a genetic anomaly that provides resistance to HIV, and it is thought that a partial form of this anomaly may lead to slower progression of the illness.

and shameful thoughts that seem totally unacceptable, and yet there they are. You may think they are so bad that you must suppress them, and that is the worst thing to do. In the long run, it is much better to admit them into consciousness, let them percolate in your mind, and see how you can analyze them yourself. Sometimes it is good to have a trusted set of colleagues, a peer supervision group or something of that nature, where you can talk about your countertransference emotions, so you can find out that what you thought was a terrible reaction is nevertheless fairly common and may ultimately be useful to the treatment.

Many of the case histories in this book describe, explicitly or implicitly, the interface of such countertransference reactions with the needs and transference reactions of the patient. This is the hallmark of the contemporary interpersonal approach to psychoanalysis. There is no such thing as purely objective listening or an objective interpretation. To be of maximum help to the patient, the psychotherapist must attend to all of her own emotional reactions to the patient, and must clarify her own personal biases when trying to formulate the direction and aims of the treatment.

I will outline just a few typical clinical situations that the psychotherapist of AIDS patients tends to face, the kinds of medical and psychological knowledge that the psychotherapist needs in each situation, and some of the possible countertransference difficulties that the therapist may have to confront.

Learning of the HIV-Positive Diagnosis

Consider the patient who has just discovered that he is HIV-positive. His T-cell count is high, his physical health seems fine, but he is having a very serious psychological reaction to the diagnosis, which may range from anxiety to panic. He may wonder, is this a death sentence? Should I end my life now, before I have to face any suffering?

It is important that the clinician be able to counsel the patient on the realities of AIDS. The patient may be told, for example, that there is great uncertainty as to the course of the illness for any individual; that it is possible for those with HIV infection but no opportunistic infections to live symptom-free for 10 years or more; that some people seem never to progress from HIV infection to AIDS as currently defined, although most people do (Buchbinder et al., 1993); that people can live with AIDS itself for 10 years or more, and that the current increased rate of medical progress is making the idea of a cure a much closer possibility; that it is possible to head off many of the opportunistic infections with prophylactic medications; and that the best strategy for living is to do those things that one wants to do as best one can for as long as one can, while making informed choices on all those issues that one can affect. It is also important to educate AIDS patients on how to be active participants in their medical care; the medical treatment of AIDS does not fit the model that many modern Westerners expect, in which the doctor diagnoses the ailment and prescribes a treatment, which, if followed faithfully, leads to cure. Instead, there are great uncertainties and gaps of knowledge about much of AIDS diagnosis, treatment, and outcome, and the patient benefits from active involvement in treatment decisions. But that strategy has to be adapted to the patient's personality style; some people prefer to let their doctors take charge, while others prefer more collaboration.

For example, a patient of mine experienced severe gastric pain. After several hospitalizations, during which his suffering was attributed to the parasite cryptosporidium, a sigmoidoscopy was performed, and he was found to have growths in his colon caused by pneumocystis carinii, which commonly causes pneumonia in AIDS patients. The physician said that this manifestation of PCP had never been reported before. Had the patient been less persistent or in a less sophisticated hospital, his ailment would probably not have been diagnosed and treated properly.

Thus, patients must learn to be educated consumers, often choosing among treatments of relative uncertainty, and often needing to advocate for themselves to obtain satisfactory medical treatment. They (and their therapists) may benefit from subscribing to one of the newsletters that discuss the latest findings about AIDS, such as *AIDS Treatment News, Treatment News: GMHC Newsletter of Experimental AIDS Therapies,* or *BETA: Bulletin of Experimental Treatments for AIDS.* Although much of the necessary information can be taught by AIDS counselors and in support groups (which may be valuable additions to any ongoing psychotherapy), the psychotherapist can be especially useful for analyzing and working with barriers to effective use of this information, including issues of passivity, wishes for caretaking, and problematic relations to authority.

Sometimes, the psychotherapist can help the patient and physician to fit their personality styles together when there is a disagreement about how to proceed medically. This may vary dramatically at different periods of the illness, and there is something of an expectable cycle. In the beginning of the illness, the physician may be idealized by the patient, and there may be great hope. Later, as the medical situation deteriorates, the idealization may break down; the doctor may be blamed for the decline in health and considered to be insensitive and no longer caring. The physician may pick up this attitude and may, perhaps unconsciously, respond to the patient's resentment as well as to his own feeling of helplessness, with a complementary withdrawal. (Much as in psychoanalysis, there is a complementarity to transference and countertransference.)

In order to intervene effectively when there is such a clash, the therapist must take into account the psychology of the physician as well as of the patient. While the variation can be very great, some general psychological principles may apply to physicians. Since physicians like to be effective, they like to be able to do something that will help the patient, and they don't like to feel helpless or have their patients die. Therefore, there may be some withdrawal from the patient when the physician feels less effective. It is important to consider whether some sort of physician burnout is going on, and whether the patient can ameliorate the situation by voicing his concerns to his physician. Sometimes, of course, the reality is that there just is not anything more that the physician can do for the patient. The physician may not have burned out, but the medical resources have.

On the other hand, some physicians want to intervene more aggressively than the patient does, and the physician may feel that the patient is being uncooperative, whereas the patient may feel that the physician is unwilling to consider dissenting opinions. There is often no clearly right answer in these situations, and either the physician or the patient or both may be very anxious in the face of uncertainty. For example, early in the illness, when patients are HIV-positive but asymptomatic, some physicians (and some patients) feel more comfortable doing something. There was a period in the late 1980s when AZT was being prescribed as soon as a patient's T cells reached 500. But some patients felt that AZT was too toxic and refused the medication against the advice of their doctors. Today, we know that they may have been right. Starting AZT that early not only did not help the patient's longevity, it could make the AZT less useful later in the illness when it was more important.

Starting in 1995, when there were new indications that a cocktail of several antivirals might be useful, the whole question of early intervention was raised again. There was the temptation among some patients to jump at the latest medical hope, and there was cynicism among other patients who thought, "I've seen this before, and I am not going to be someone's guinea pig." The balance between the two views is the individual's decision. The psychotherapist should be as informed as possible about the latest findings and treatments, so that he can engage the patient in a fruitful exploration of the psychological issues involved, without directing the patient's decision.[4] Some patients are inclined to avoid most aggressive medicine, whereas others are most comfortable with an all-out attack, and there are many who are in between on this continuum.

Some patients avail themselves of a range of "alternative" medical treatments. These can include homeopathic remedies, massage, holistic practices of bodily cleansing, shamanistic exercises, nutritional regimens, and imaging techniques. The possibilities are quite a bit more extensive (see Abrams, 1990, 1992; Greenberg, 1994; McCutchan, 1994). Most of these treatments are of unproven effectiveness. They usually do no harm, and they sometimes bring on physical improvements. Whether this is due to a placebo effect is not always clear, but placebo effects can be powerful. Psychotherapists should remain open-minded about such alternative treatments, especially as long as there is no definitive cure for AIDS. Therapists may feel more conflicted if the patient refuses traditional medicine even while facing serious medical setbacks. Psychotherapists need to feel free to discuss these issues openly with their patients, keeping in mind that the patient has ultimate responsibility for his or her own life.[5]

After the Initial Diagnosis

Once a patient has stabilized and resolved the initial panic reaction to the HIV-positive diagnosis, he may engage in the whole range of psychotherapeutic efforts. I have seen quite a few patients bring about unusually rapid and profound characterological changes and accomplish life goals in a few years that they had been putting off for decades. It had already been observed that reaching middle age and getting closer to feelings of mortality enabled some very resistant patients to make good use of psychotherapy (Kernberg, 1980; King, 1980; Myers, 1987). Now we are observing that people of all ages, when confronted with mortality, can do the same thing. I have worked with blocked writers who published

4. The principles of this sort of psychotherapeutic intervention applies to any other medical decision where there is a real balance between risk and benefit. For example, the question may come up about whether to surgically remove a precancerous but nonmalignant tumor, or whether, in a pregnancy, to have an amniocentesis. The patient may be told the statistical likelihood of a negative outcome of either choice, but the numbers are not useful without an exploration of the *psychological* valences of the two choices.

5. See chapters by Drs. Shapiro and Petrucelli. Shapiro describes a patient who avoided nearly all traditional Western medicine and the psychotherapist's changing countertransference reactions to this treatment strategy over time.

several books. People who had spent most of their lives single formed committed and loving relationships. Some people managed to make peace with estranged family members and confront parental homophobia and other prejudices. Some people who had lived marginal lives of poverty, drugs, and aimlessness found themselves clearing their systems of drugs and being able to restructure their lives with great drive and intensity of purpose. And some AIDS patients from deprived backgrounds who made their way into some of the better treatment programs found that they were being given close and caring professional attention, the likes of which they had never received in their lifetimes.

The pressure of time often leads patients to confront character resistances much more forcefully and efficiently, so that impressive progress can often be made, and major life changes that the patient has always desired can at times be realized under "time-pressure psychoanalysis." This may be related to the old technique of setting an arbitrary termination date to an analysis, as discussed by Freud (1918, 1937) and Ferenczi and Rank (1923).

Working with AIDS for over 15 years has had slow, subtle, but very significant effects on my clinical work, which I think may teach all of us who do psychotherapy some important lessons. Sandor Ferenczi once wrote a paper on the elasticity of psychoanalytic technique. I think that working with people with AIDS for 15 years has taught me a level of elasticity beyond what I ever thought could work within a psychoanalytic framework.

As psychotherapists, we often consider a gradient between interpreting with insights that would benefit the patient and respecting the tenacity of the patient's defenses and his tolerable level of anxiety. In working with an HIV-infected patient whose life is likely to be cut short, the choice between interpreting and supporting defenses takes on a heightened urgency. One might offer insights more rapidly, even if it increases the risk that the patient's anxiety level will be much higher. On the other hand, one might be inclined to be primarily supportive and not to interpret so vigorously, perhaps judging the patient's state as too precarious to tolerate much anxiety. The choice must take into account the patient's wishes and be informed by clinical judgment.

For example, a middle-aged man came to me for analysis. He was HIV-positive but still asymptomatic. He had been in analysis previously for many years, yet a severely pathological character structure was still in place. He was immensely controlling, which alienated most of his prospects for romance. At the same time, he was extremely ingratiating and masochistic with persons in authority; this led to a much-repeated pattern of their abusing him, and of his then feeling victimized and seeking retribution.

He asked for a "pressure-cooker analysis." Although we analyzed the masochistic aspects of this wish, it had enough of a real practicality to be attempted, while being always alert to the risks of recreating his familiar pattern of abusive relationships. I found myself making interpretations to this man that rocked his equilibrium.

Between sessions I often worried: "That was too much for him; he'll never come back." I recognized, with some difficulty, that my thought that he would not return might have a wishful aspect, signifying my despair at whether he could emerge from his neurotic whirlpool and have some good years before the inevitable terminal illness made it too late. There were a few stormy interruptions, but he stayed with the analysis in the long run and met my interpretive challenges with his own determination. There were some important character changes, certainly not complete, but substantial enough to allow him to regain some professional productivity and happiness in a personal relationship. I do not know if I would have worked at this pace had he not been HIV-positive, or if he would have tolerated such work had he not been HIV-positive.

In working with AIDS patients, as with all severely ill patients, there is a heightened necessity for taking account of and analyzing the countertransference. Fears of contagion are as common as they are irrational, and must be mastered. I don't know of any HIV-negative psychotherapist working with AIDS patients who has not had at least a fleeting fear about contagion, whether from touching the doorknob that the patient has touched, using the same bathroom, or from some other means, no matter how strong the evidence that such contagion does not occur. The psychotherapist can use such fearful fantasies to gain empathy with the dread that the patient's loved ones may be experiencing, but such reactions are best examined privately, if possible; AIDS patients experience enough dread and self-loathing without getting any additional burdens from the analyst (Schaffner, 1990, 1994; Walker, 1991). Blaming the patient for the illness, whether as an attempt to distance oneself from the danger of illness or because of judgmental attitudes about homosexuality and drug use, is an especially destructive countertransference trend in work with AIDS patients.

Timing of Interpretations

One of the lessons of my work with AIDS patients, which may be useful to all of us who do psychotherapy, has to do with our sense of time and the timing of our interpretations. Many of us are familiar with the old principle of interpretation that says, "Make an interpretation at the point that the patient is on the verge of having the realization himself." This may have seemed a valid principle when patients were often seen five times a week, were young, and had a normal life span ahead of them. It certainly guarded against undue anxiety that might frighten the patient or drive her prematurely from treatment.

Working with AIDS has changed my view of that principle. If I have a clear formulation in mind of what the focal issue is for the patient, I would prefer to state it as soon as possible. The question is less of when than of how. How can I say what I have formulated in such a way that the patient will at least hear it with minimal anxiety, or with sufficiently low anxiety to be able to consider it and work with it?[6]

I worked with one gay man with AIDS, an attorney in his early 40s, who had always been single and earnestly desired to develop a committed relationship. His view of how that relationship would go was quite clear and detailed, which at first seemed helpful to me. I thought I was clear about what he wanted. But as I worked with him, he began a few relationships that were ended abruptly by the other person. I came to realize that his view of how a relationship should go was so fixed that he was not always taking into account what the other person wanted. He was intent on fulfilling what he called his "project for the next decade," but he sometimes missed clues that the other person felt pushed into a style of relatedness with which he did not feel comfortable.

I was reminded of the Greek myth of Procrustes. As Robert Graves (1955) tells us, in one version of the myth, "Procrustes lived beside the

---

6. In my view, Freud happened on a fascinating strategy for making difficult interpretations palatable. That is, he related the patient's life situation to one in mythology or in fiction. Freud did this brilliantly with the Oedipus complex. Of course, some of us now doubt that the Oedipus complex is a universal phenomenon. Several people have also pointed out how Freud misunderstood or distorted the Oedipus myth in order to formulate his complex (e.g., Garber, 1995). But in my view, the genius of the Oedipus complex is that it allowed Freud to identify a dynamic in people that most would not want to consider about themselves—namely, murderous wishes toward one's father and sexual desires towards one's mother, or vice versa. In Freud's early days, it would have been shocking, as well as a blow to one's self-esteem, to have such base desires. But to say, as Freud did, you have feelings that are in tune with one of the great mythological characters in history served a double purpose of getting people intrigued with the grandeur of these seemingly base desires. It also boosted their self-esteem, even as they heard this bad news, to think of themselves identified with one of the grand figures of mythological history, who, for all his faults, was possessed of great powers that included solving the riddle of the Sphinx.

Others have since followed in Freud's footsteps, naming complexes and syndromes after mythical figures, for instance, Maslow's (1967) description of the Jonah syndrome, which is an evasion of one's highest possibilities in life by hiding, as Jonah tried to do (p. 163).

road and had one bed in his house. Offering a night's lodging to travelers, he would lengthen or shorten the traveler to fit the bed. If they were too tall for the bed, he would saw off as much of their legs as projected beyond it" (pp. 329–330). I told the patient that he was like Procrustes. He tried to fit everyone into his "project for the next decade," and he balked when they didn't fit. Psychoanalytic cure for Procrustes might have been to learn to adjust his bed to his guests, rather than the other way around, and so it was for this patient. The aim in therapy became for him to have insight into this and to enable himself to be more flexible. He did so, and was able to develop a very serious, committed relationship.

The subject of dating often brings up the difficult question of when to tell the prospective partner that one is HIV-positive. Many patients fear that if they tell someone right away that they are HIV-positive, the other person will inevitably reject them as a romantic partner. On the other hand, if the patient hides the fact that he is HIV-positive, when the partner does find out, he is likely to feel betrayed, and so the prospects of continuing the relationship will be dismal. This is a very difficult situation, being "between a rock and a hard place," and the psychotherapist often must help the single HIV-positive patient to find his or her way through this situation, which interacts with characterological issues. Usually, the best teacher is experience. Green (1989) believes that most people who are HIV-negative, especially if heterosexual, would not consider having a sexual relationship with someone who is HIV-positive. Such rejection certainly does occur; Bayer (1989) writes eloquently about the rejection he experienced trying to date as a single hemophiliac with HIV. But such rejection is not always the rule. Some people with AIDS have found loving partners who are HIV-negative.[7]

The Choice of Which Issues to Work On

In psychotherapy, we often have to consider whether certain forms of character pathology are adaptive for a particular patient. In working with people with AIDS, one makes the judgment to leave alone certain character traits that one would probably deal with in psychotherapy with a physically healthy patient. I worked with someone who was very exploitive and deceptive. He came to me for psychotherapy, without having adequate medical treatment in place. Part of his difficulties had to do with his personality. I helped him take care of these issues.

7. See chapter by Dr. Shapiro for the case of a woman with AIDS who married an HIV-negative man.

After I had helped him, he let me know that he had been seeing two other psychotherapists concurrently, plus he was in a psychotherapy-medication study. He felt he hadn't wanted to let me know about these other treatments until I had proven myself to him. This sort of exploitation was pervasive in his life, and I noted it matter-of-factly to him. But I realized that this sort of exploitiveness was also functional with his illness; had he not had AIDS, I would have dealt with this character issue much more forcefully.[8]

AIDS can take on very different personal meanings for each individual and, often, conflicting meanings may reside in the same individual (Schwartzberg, 1993). For example, many gay men who are HIV-positive experience a new sense of belonging. As one man told Schwartzberg,

> There's going to be a lot of positive stuff that comes out of this. Gay people can now say "We" as a people in a way that we couldn't before this happened. . . . For me, the meaning of AIDS is going to be a lot of maturity on the part of the gay community. We're going to be healthier as a community than we were before. We're going to be more concerned about each other, and taking our lives as gay people more seriously [p. 485].

Yet Schwartzberg also found that many of the same men now found that HIV at times made them feel isolated from others who were HIV-negative, as shown in this quotation.

> A good friend telephoned me recently with the results of his test. He's negative. Don't misunderstand—I was overjoyed for him. But I also felt something had come between us, a wall, and things will never be quite the same between us. I wanted to say to him, 'I know how you feel,' but I couldn't, because I don't [p. 486].

Schwartzberg (1994) identifies four basic kinds of meaning-making among people with HIV: (1) high meaning; (2) defensive meaning; (3) shattered meaning; and (4) irrelevant meaning. The latter group (about one in five of Schwartzberg's sample) may be the most difficult for the psychotherapist—people who feel that HIV has had no particular significant effect, positive or negative, on their lives. As one man put it, "My day-to-day life has not been much affected. I don't detect any real change in who I am as a person, other than opening me up a bit more . . . I carry on a normal life. . . . A lot of people say you use your time better, but I'm not sure you do. . . . Overall, it hasn't changed my view too much" (p. 488).

8. See chapters by Drs. Gartner and Mujica for similar clinical dilemmas.

Such people may seek psychotherapy for support with very concrete problems faced in dealing with HIV. The psychotherapist who is accustomed to analyzing and creating meaning with his patients may feel stymied by such a patient. He should accept the circumscribed goals of the patient for as long as necessary, or refer the patient to someone who can.

Of course, the lack of psychological-mindedness or interest in personal meaning may change over time. Consider Jay, a highly schizoid man of 42, who had had AIDS for three years when he first consulted me. He presented at the initial interview as if he had no interests and no feelings. "What can therapy do for me?" he asked me. He was generally unresponsive to any interpretations, and I wondered if I could be of any help to him. And yet, despite his apparent apathy and lack of a stated goal, he was there, in my office, so I presumed he wanted something from therapy, and I agreed to work with him.

Our initial work was focused on his complaints about the medical care he was receiving. I helped him find an alternative physician as well as a support group. His self-esteem was almost totally invested in his personal appearance. When he started to develop KS lesions on his face, I helped him find ways to have them removed. He seemed uninterested in restructuring his personality, but I knew it was only a matter of time before his personal appearance would deteriorate beyond his control, and there might be great despair.

He had a "lover," Alex, with whom he worked in business part-time. The way Jay described the relationship sounded exploitive; Alex would cook for Jay and take care of him when necessary; but Jay mostly liked to live alone, and only stayed at Alex's house when he needed caretaking. Given the possibly short amount of time he had left, I had to wonder: Is my therapeutic aim to help him get involved in a more giving, mutual relationship or to maintain his steady supply of caretaking? It is important in such a case to find out what the patient's stated goals are; he seemed to want to keep the status quo in that area for now. And I recognized that there was much about him I didn't know.

Four months into treatment, he acknowledged a yearning for physical contact. He was having no sexual relationship, with Alex or anyone else. He brought up his romantic history. He had always been gay, and the one person with whom he had been seriously in love, he cheated on constantly. Thereafter, his relationships took on a constant cast of mutual infidelity.

I then discovered that his parents' marriage had been one of people "living together separately." His father had a mistress, but stayed for a number of years with his wife after she found out. Later they separated, but never divorced. When I wondered whether this had anything to do with Jay's own pattern of relationships, he said, flat out, "I can't see how the two could have anything to do with one another."

But the seed was planted in his thinking. Three weeks later, this man, who had refused any genetic interpretation of his fear of closeness, started analyzing his lover's fear of closeness, based on his history! This was an important stage in his therapy. He was able to try out interpretations about another person that were relevant to himself, what I have called "projective interpretation" (Blechner, 1992, 1996).

Psychotherapy with Patients in Late-Stage AIDS

Some patients may come to the psychotherapist for the first time when they are already in the late stages of AIDS. Often, they are referred by the physician, who identifies a serious depression that does not respond to medication alone. Patients who come for therapy in this situation are often having great difficulty confronting the changes in their experience of life, and they may be having a different kind of panic—the panic of uncertain but close mortality. Such patients are not likely to be interested in fundamental character change; they are more likely to be seeking support. I should say that good supportive psychotherapy is at least as difficult to do as good exploratory psychotherapy. It requires that you always stay close to the emotional situation of the patient in the moment. A patient who is in deep despair about a medical setback does not need confrontation; he needs empathy, with perhaps a gentle reminder of previous times when his medical condition got worse and then was turned around. For many patients, it is not death itself that is feared, but intractable pain and the loss of functioning and mobility. Especially difficult is blindness caused by cytomegalovirus infection, persistent pain in the extremities from neuropathy, drastic loss of weight and bowel control, and AIDS dementia. The therapist may find herself needed for some unusual functions with the demented patient, including collaborating with the patient in fantasizing about a hopeful future that the therapist knows is not possible.[9]

It is very common for patients to form the fantasy during psychotherapy that the psychotherapist will somehow be able to cure the AIDS. Most therapists have also had such fantasies. Studies have shown that psychological treatment increases the average survival time of people with different kinds of cancer (e.g., Spiegel et al., 1989; Fawzy et al.,

9. See the chapter by Dr. Marisak for a description of such a therapeutic relationship and the countertransference difficulties it may raise.

1993), and it may well be true of AIDS. But while survival time may increase, I have never seen psychological treatment cure anyone of AIDS.

A patient with advanced AIDS told me that when he was a teenager, he was severely ill for four years and seemed near death. The doctors were confused, but finally a specialist determined that he had a very rare illness, which was curable. He was then properly treated and recovered. So he had great trust in Western medicine but believed that the patient had to stay one step ahead of the physician.

This adolescent experience shaped his approach to having AIDS as an adult. He read medical textbooks constantly and often impressed his physicians with his knowledge. I saw him question a planned intervention more than once, and ultimately prove that he was right. When he said to me, "The doctors thought I was supposed to die two years ago, and yet here I am; I think I will be the first one to beat this thing," I noticed myself thinking, "I know it has never happened, and it probably will not, but maybe. . . ." Unfortunately, when it started to look like his death was inevitable, I became very depressed. These fantasies of rescue have a great function in maintaining enthusiasm in both the patient and the therapist, but if you believe them too much, you may burn out.

Loneliness

One of the most serious problems of patients in the late stages of AIDS may be extreme loneliness. Some may have been abandoned by family or friends, but loneliness can occur even when there is an apparently large personal network. The loneliness may come when his caregivers start to panic about their own mortality and to keep a certain distance from his experience. Also, women with AIDS often feel required to maintain their role in supporting their family's functioning, so that they try to hide their physical and psychological distress from family members, which makes them feel even more lonely. One woman with AIDS described her situation in this way (Dansky, 1994):

> There was this friend over the other day, and he's talkin' to Herbie about women, that they're different now. I just thinkin' about my doin' the laundry after a D and C and carryin' it up five flights of stairs. And moppin' the floor. And givin' Herbie his AZT, and goin' to the clinic for me. Ya know what I mean? And this prick is talkin' about women. What am I supposed to be: supermom and superwife? [p. 223].

For some patients, the hardest and loneliest times are periods of relative health *after* a serious hospitalization. A patient of mine was hospitalized with AIDS for over two months, with five difficult-to-treat infections. He had an extraordinary set of friends and relatives who visited him and cared for him round the clock. I myself visited him in the hospital once a week, and more often during a period when he was psychotic. We had sessions in his hospital room, and in one session I thought he would die in front of my eyes.

But he didn't. As happens not infrequently, people in late stages of AIDS are given up for lost, and then they rebound. The postrebound period can be very difficult. The patient was eventually discharged from the hospital, regained the weight he had lost, and looked quite healthy. Suddenly, the tremendous support network that had surrounded him in the hospital thinned out, and he felt lonely, rejected, and depressed. He spoke nostalgically of his time in the hospital, of the peak emotional experiences he had had. His early life had been one of the most deprived I have ever heard of. He and his five siblings had been abandoned by both parents for a year and lived by begging, stealing, and living in unoccupied dwellings. It was useful in psychotherapy that we clarified the patterns of abandonment that he had grown used to in his childhood, and which he tended to accept passively, so that he could change now and actively talk to his friends and relatives about his isolation.

The Role of the Psychotherapist

It is not unusual for psychotherapists to abandon their roles with AIDS patients and to get directly involved in their patients' lives. One of the assistants of Kübler-Ross (1987) has described her total personal involvement and commitment to a dying patient. It reminds one of Sechehaye's (1951) extraordinary devotion to her schizophrenic patient, Renée, which led to great therapeutic gains, but could not become a general method of working because of the enormous demands put on the therapist's time and energy; such limitless devotion would quickly lead to burnout. While AIDS patients often need extraordinary caregiving, there is a good case to be made for the psychotherapist to maintain his therapeutically neutral position, while other caregivers meet the other needs of the patient.[10] This situation allows the patient to bring his most painful and destructive fantasies and emotions to the therapist, like

10. See chapter by Dr. Eisold for an example of a therapist's experiences leading her to change her view on this issue.

wanting to kill the person who gave him AIDS, or to kill people who don't have HIV and who stigmatize those who do and treat them badly. The sessions can then function as a kind of crucible for these unmentionable feelings, which allows the patient to carry on productively outside the sessions. If the patient actually needs the psychotherapist for caregiving outside the sessions, this crucial function of the psychotherapist is compromised. But the psychotherapist must be sure that the AIDS patient has set up such an independent support network.

For example, I worked with a gay couple, Allen and Bill, who started treatment shortly after Bill was diagnosed with AIDS. Allen was HIV-negative. They stayed in treatment for nearly three years, not too long before Bill died. Both were also in individual therapy, and as Bill became more ill, his individual therapist stepped out of role considerably, in very nurturant ways about which Allen and Bill were ambivalent.

There was one couple's session in which Allen complained of Bill's lack of responsiveness and accused him of hiding his real feelings. Just before the end of the session, Bill burst out in a rage that yes, he was furious and was beset by fantasies of murdering people who do not have AIDS, and could anyone understand that? I was dumbstruck by his outburst and could say nothing. It felt in some way relieving that he had himself acknowledged the personal terror that he was experiencing. But I also felt guilty that I had been unable to speak. I thought, they will never come back after that. This was one of many, many fantasies of their stopping treatment that I gradually came to realize were part of my own wish not to have to face the terrible things that were to come.

But they did come back the next week. Relations between them had improved dramatically since the previous session, and both seemed in good spirits. They referred to the previous session as "the voodoo session" and were grateful for it.

The Task of the Psychotherapist

A therapist needs to help all AIDS patients make peace with the lives they have lived. What has the patient done of value? How has he lived? Why did he make the choices that he did? At times, there is a need to resolve long-standing conflicts, to settle old scores, or to right certain wrongs. The patient may want to make reparation to someone he has wronged, to thank someone who has been important, to admonish or cut off someone who has treated him badly. This does not mean that with such patients an exploration of the early history is irrelevant. On the contrary, sometimes an exploration of the past, with a few pointed interpretations, may clarify, for a patient who has never before been in psychotherapy, how he came to live life as he did. This can sometimes be done effectively in just a few sessions, even in just one or two consultations.

For example, a man in the late stages of AIDS came to me because he was having very severe nightmares. As we explored the content of his dreams, it was clear that there were unresolved conflicts with his family, mainly about his always having to be the strong person supporting the other members of the family, a position that was especially painful now that he had AIDS. He got the courage to bring this up with his family and had some very difficult and revealing discussions with them. And then the nightmares stopped.

AIDS has taught us to deal psychoanalytically with a greatly expanded range of problems. Some of these issues are quite new, and some, while always present, are difficult topics that many of us avoid as much as possible. Death and mortality are probably the most difficult for us. Most of us avoid thinking about our own death, and many of us superstitiously avoid doing anything related to death, like writing a will. Yet for someone who has AIDS, it is very important at least to make preparations, like a will and a health-care proxy. I have seen some therapists in supervision who have had to confront their own countertransference squeamishness about death and mortality before they could address this issue with their patients.

Kübler-Ross (1969) has provided a model for facing a terminal illness, with five sequential stages: denial, anger, bargaining, depression, and acceptance. While patients may have all of these experiences, they may occur in a different order and not necessarily as separate entities. Theoretical models of death and dying may be of some use in conceptualizing the experience, although they are no substitute for continual self-examination of one's own experience of health, dying, and of the priorities of living and potential blocks to empathy.[11] It is useful for the psychotherapist to read psychologically aware first-person accounts of people with AIDS (e.g., Rowland, 1988; Callen, 1991; Monette, 1994).

Some psychotherapists deal with their fear of death by a counterphobic strategy. They try compulsively to get their patients to talk about death, with a kind of fake bravado, even at a time when the patient has other concerns. This countertransference reaction is usually not very helpful to patients. In a similar vein, I once worked with an HIV-positive man whose previous therapist had interpreted every dream in terms of HIV, which at times required a real stretch of the imagination. This is

11. See chapters by Drs. Eisold and Gartner for examples of therapists simultaneously tracking their patients' and their own reactions to death.

another dangerous countertransference distortion; we have to remember that a person with HIV is still a person, with all kinds of psychological issues besides HIV.

Bereavement

One of the continual themes that comes up with AIDS patients and with those who are close to them is bereavement. There is great sadness in losing someone to AIDS; the deterioration is horrible to watch, more so if you love the person who is dying; often, after the illness has progressed for a long time, one wishes consciously or unconsciously for the person's death, and this can evoke great guilt. These and related phenomena are all familiar to people who have cared for and lost loved ones to other slow, painful, and disfiguring diseases, like cancer (Eissler, 1955; Kübler-Ross, 1969; Adler et al., 1975).

Loss makes one keenly aware of the reality of what psychoanalysts call "object relations." Object relations theory proposes that we retain a mental representation of every person we know or have known, which may be different in some respects from the actual person (as perceived by others) and can persist if the person leaves or dies. We also maintain a mental representation of ourselves, and of ourselves in relation to the other person. So interpersonal relations have a life of their own in the mind of each of us, and even if the other person dies, our relationship with him can survive and continue in our minds (or brains, or souls, as you wish). We know how common it is for people to speak to the deceased in cemeteries; but our relations with the deceased can continue and change for as long as we survive them. In that sense there is a *psychic* afterlife; the relationship can and does continue even when one person dies. You may conjure up the dead person at will, see her, hear her, smell her, as if she were still with you, which, psychologically speaking, she is.

I have on my shelf several books written by patients who have died of AIDS. I can pick up a book and a flood of memories about its author comes rushing back: the first session, the hard sessions, and the rageful sessions; the dreams we interpreted together, the breakthroughs, and the gratifying progress; the shift from relatively unobtrusive HIV-infection into serious illness; the dread, the pain, the suffering, the decline, the death, the mourning, the remembering.

The better you understand your own way of dealing with grief and loss, the better you will be able to help others deal with their own grief. Patients may come to psychotherapy because of difficulties grieving the loss of a loved one. The source of difficulty can vary enormously, including unresolved guilt about the caretaking during the illness, unconscious ambivalence about the deceased, and a complex pattern of projection, introjection, and identification with aspects of the deceased (Szalita, 1974). The psychotherapist must be alert to the experience of the patient before the loved one's illness and to the nature of the relationship.

For example, Hal was a choreographer in his mid-40s who had been partners with a man, Gary, for 21 years. They were partners in every sense of the word: they were romantic lovers, they lived together, and they worked together in a very successful professional collaboration. When Gary died of AIDS, there was an elaborate funeral. Hal became severely depressed and suicidal and was referred to me for psychotherapy. A number of causes of the depression emerged.

For one thing, Hal had formed a symbiotic bond with Gary in their work life and was unsure of his ability to continue to be productive in their field. There was a need to work out the loss of Gary as a person, and to distinguish it from the experienced loss of a part of Hal himself that had become identified with Gary (as outlined by Freud, 1917). As the therapy progressed, Hal not only was able to thrive professionally, but found that, on his own, he took his work in new directions. This development was gratifying, but it also induced guilt for proceeding without Gary.

Hal had hallucinations, seeing himself hung from a butcher's hook. These were traced back to an early history, which he had partially repressed, of being severely beaten by his older brothers. Recovering the profundity of these early traumata brought to light some of the unconscious reasons for Hal's fearfulness in facing life alone, without Gary.

Hal and Gary had never articulated the nature of their relationship to Hal's parents, although the parents had stayed in their home and had seen that they shared a bedroom. When Gary died, Hal's parents took no notice of it and did not attend the funeral. The analysis of this experience brought to light a severe, internalized homophobia in Hal, along with a rage reaction at his parents' lack of concern or acknowledgment of the relationship.

This is a common problem among gay men who lose a partner to AIDS. In Hal's case, there was at least a well-worked-out will that allowed for an orderly inheritance of their joint assets. It is unfortunately quite common for gay men to die without a will, in which case the law requires that all the assets be left to the next of kin, usually the parents or another close blood relative. There are many situations in which partners of gay men are evicted from the homes that they shared with the deceased partner, even though they may have contributed financially to the home. When the parents of the deceased partner are not respectful of the relationship, there can be very ugly sequelae. But even if they have been respectful of the relationship before their son's death, they may shift their attitude after the death, irrationally blaming the partner for their son's homosexuality or his having AIDS. I know of one case where the parents sued the partner to get not only their home and joint financial assets but the deceased's old clothes. The therapist must be sensitive to the grossly traumatic nature of such situations, as well as be alert to the ways that the survivor may accept such injustices and subsequently attack himself unconsciously.

It is important for psychotherapists to know that hallucinations, in which the survivor sees the dead person who is missed, are quite common. A study of widows and widowers found that about 50 percent experienced hallucinations of their late spouses (Rees, 1975; see also Marris, 1958; Yamamoto et al., 1969). These kinds of hallucinations are significant not only because of their ordinariness but because of their emotional quality. The survivor sees the dead person and experiences this without any particular anxiety, almost as if it were a matter-of-fact occurrence, even though she is aware that it is hallucination. A widow may be sitting in her living room and suddenly see her late husband sitting in his customary favorite chair. She may even speak with him and hear his response. These experiences often help in the mourning process and are not indicative of a schizophrenic process.

Interestingly, while Hal had a history of anxiety-filled hallucinations, he later had this kind of nonanxious, soothing hallucination of the return of the dead. He was riding his bicycle (a sport that he had begun after Gary's death) and suddenly saw Gary riding along next to him (Gary had never ridden a bicycle during his lifetime). Hal felt comforted by seeing Gary with him; it indicated to him that Gary was now integrated into his new life. He knew it was a hallucination, although sensorially it felt totally real. During the weeks that followed this hallucination, Hal was able to engage in a number of social interactions that signaled a new freedom and a healing of his loss.

Massive Bereavement and Repeated Survivors

A new and special problem with AIDS that has become more common in recent years is what I have called "massive bereavement" (Blechner, 1993a). Because AIDS has until now been especially concentrated among certain groups, members of those groups have had to face losing many or all of their loved ones and acquaintances. Some keep lists, and their losses can number more than 100. The longer the epidemic goes on, the more common is this syndrome, and the more severe. I have heard quite a few gay men claim that they have lost all of their friends to the disease. Such experiences have until now been rare in our society, with certain exceptions, such as people who have lost their entire families in wartime or through the Holocaust. I think of such people as "repeated survivors." Over and over, they have succumbed to loss. Psychotherapy with such AIDS survivors is especially difficult because the trauma is not over; repeated survivors cannot set aside the past and make a new beginning because the AIDS epidemic still looms large; many fear that they will start new relationships and that those, too, may succumb to AIDS (Goldman, 1989). Like the survivors of the Black Death of the Middle Ages, everyone has to find his or her own way of coping with the great losses of the past and the dread of future losses. Boccaccio (1353) wrote about the Black Death in *The Decameron*, and his observations are eerily relevant to us today:

> the number of deaths reported in the city whether by day or night was so enormous that it astonished all who heard tell of it, to say nothing of the people who actually witnessed the carnage. And it was perhaps inevitable that among the citizens who survived there arose certain customs that were quite contrary to established tradition [p. 54].

Six hundred years after Boccaccio wrote this, survivors of the AIDS epidemic are having to find their own customs and rituals, contrary to established tradition, to deal with massive bereavement and to find a way of going on with their lives. For example, I worked with a gay man in his 30s who had had three lovers die of AIDS, and the man he was currently dating had just revealed that he was HIV-positive. This man, who was still HIV-negative, felt extreme grief and had made concrete plans for suicide. I raised the question whether he, personally, could have another relationship with someone who is HIV-positive; clearly his own life was at risk, more from suicide than from HIV, and he had to respect his limitations.

I saw another man in treatment who had had a brief period of hallucinations and delusions, which lasted for a few days. He was in his mid-70s, gay, and had been single all his life. He lived alone and had lost most of his friends to AIDS. His closest friend, Bill, who was his only remaining steady human contact, now had late-stage AIDS. One day he came home and hallucinated that his small apartment was filled with mimes in whiteface. When he tried to talk to them, they wouldn't respond. Then he looked and saw his close friend Bill lying in his bed with the covers over his head. As I listened to his history, it seemed probable that the psychotic experiences had been triggered by a new medication that he had started; they did, in fact, stop when the medication was discontinued. But the content of the hallucinations was important; all the different hallucinations involved large crowds of people arriving unannounced. His hallucinations were like wish-fulfillment dreams or like the end of the movie *Longtime Companion,* in which the thousands of people who have died of AIDS return. They highlighted his current loneliness, and his dread of the even greater loneliness to come when Bill would die. Psychotherapy helped him address this anxiety-laden future.

Repeated survivors experience survivor guilt and depression, but they also cope with such experiences through unique defenses. For example, I worked with a gay man with AIDS, Dan, who worked with Roy, his friend and business partner. Both of them were repeated survivors. Roy had lost all of his friends to AIDS, with the exception of Dan. Roy's way of managing Dan's illness was primarily through denial. Their mutual business required extraordinary hands-on efforts, lasting for 12 hours at a stretch, in crowded circumstances that exposed Dan to multiple pathogens. Twice, after such work days, Dan ended up in the hospital. Yet Roy continued to pressure him to work; in so doing, he tried to deny that the last of his friends was dying. As the therapist, I realized that it was useless merely to discuss with Dan the wisdom of stopping this kind of work. Much more relevant was working through the blocks in communication with Roy—their mutual rage and helplessness—so that they could then resolve the practical issues themselves.

Bereavement is also a countertransference problem for the psychotherapist. Having worked with many AIDS patients for more than 15 years, I have come to observe in myself certain ways of "getting used to" AIDS that are disturbing to me. For example, I visited a patient in the hospital. He had been on vacation for three weeks, and while away, he had suddenly become severely ill. He could retain neither food nor liquid, and when he called me from the hospital, he told me he had lost a lot of weight and was very run down. I visited him in the hospital, and when I first saw him, my private thought was, "He doesn't look so bad." I found this thought upsetting; I am sure most people would have found his appearance alarming. His KS lesions were spread over his face, he was gaunt, and his skin color was rather gray. I realized how accustomed I had become to such an appearance. In fact, more than once in recent years, when a new patient who is HIV-positive but asymptomatic has come to me for consultation, I have found myself imagining that patient's appearance in the latter stages of AIDS. I have taken this partly as a self-warning, to be careful not to become overloaded with grief and burnout. (See also Shernoff, 1991.)

Parallels with the Holocaust seem inevitable. More than one account from Auschwitz talks of the so-called Moslems, the people in the camp who had undergone severe starvation and had reached a stage of deterioration in which their shuffling gait and gaunt appearance indicated, without doubt, that they would soon die. For concentration camp inmates, watching such deterioration became an everyday occurrence, and they coined the sardonic name "Moslems" to help them deal with unbearable grief and horror.

The AIDS epidemic seemed at first too horrible to approach with humor, but that has changed. An "AIDS farce" has been produced in New York, and other comic treatments of the subject have also appeared. That this has occurred and is acceptable suggests how extreme the devastation of AIDS has become, overloading the ego defenses of denial and isolation and requiring humor and different kinds of reaction formation.

Denial and reaction formation also may make their appearance in patients' dreams. For example, a man who had advanced AIDS reported this dream. "There is a piece of pink medical equipment with tubes coming out of it. My friend Neal was there. There were other people there, laughing and playing with the stupid medical equipment. We were sucking on the tubes or blowing on them. None of the people in the dream had AIDS. They all did not have AIDS."

The statement "They all did not have AIDS" contradicted the fact that the patient himself had AIDS, and that he was in the dream. In associating to the dream, he saw the dream as making light of the dreadful medical equipment that AIDS patients have to confront. The machine was pink, a color symbolizing the gay liberation movement. Neal was an HIV-negative gay man who had a wonderful sense of humor. The dream combined the medical reality of AIDS with a kind of group sex play that might have been more easygoing before AIDS. The patient was aware of the denial and reaction formation going on in the dream, but he saw them as adaptive; his capacity for cheeriness helped him to get through many difficult times and to maintain a circle of devoted friends.

The kind of splitting shown in this dream may also appear in therapists of AIDS patients. Some who have been overloaded with grief may take a consciously spartan or anesthetized stance to cover over their grief. The resulting split in the ego can be risky. If it becomes too pronounced, the therapist may act out his grief, perhaps by withdrawing from his patient. At such times, the therapist's dreams can be especially useful for clarifying both sides of the conflict. For example, I saw a man in psychotherapy who was himself a therapist working exclusively with AIDS patients. He reported this brief dream:

"I went to the memorial service of a patient who had died of AIDS. They are showing a moving picture of this man when he was healthy and mobile." He then provided these associations to the dream. "The patient had been in a wheelchair before he died. I don't remember feeling much during the dream. This patient was referred by a close friend who was his physical therapist. I had been speaking to this friend on the phone. He had been on sabbatical. I told him, jokingly, 'You went on your sabbatical and the man died.'"

The therapist told me that he didn't remember feeling much during the dream. But then we noted the punning *moving picture* that he sees in the dream. Moving picture is another term for film, but it is also an *emotionally* moving picture. The dream and his conscious associations showed the split between feeling and not feeling. Also, he blames his friend's abandonment of the patient, by going away on sabbatical, for the patient's death, which seems to absolve him of any guilt.

Of course, the dream also had personal significance for the dreamer aside from his clinical work. Although he was HIV-negative, he was often wistful about a time in the past when he was more mobile, active, and alive. He defended against this grief as well as his grief about his patient. In fact, analyzing these parallel griefs allowed my patient to separate the rational aspects of his grief from his own depression and unconscious identification with the deceased man.

If a therapist overloaded with grief does start to act out and withdraw from his patients, dreams may function as a kind of wake-up call. For example, a therapist in treatment with me reported the following dream. "I was with a dog, I think it was Scooter (the dog I grew up with as a child). There was a terrible wind blowing outside. And we were going to go out this door. As I was approaching the door, Scooter was rising up, like there was something happening to him from the air pressure. I was trying to hold him back. He started biting my hand. I couldn't tell if he wanted to go out. If we tried to take him on the subway, we'd probably miss some trains, because he'd probably be afraid to get on, but that's what we probably should do."

He then analyzed the dream himself. "The dream wasn't obviously about AIDS, but I woke up from it thinking about one of my patients with AIDS. I didn't take care of him right in the last few days. I was supposed to call his physician, and I didn't.

"It has to do with my dog Scooter's death. I know it may sound trivial, but I have always felt guilty about his death. I was away at college when he died. He needed surgery, and my parents had to take care of him. In the dream he bites me. He is angry at me for not taking care of him right. The whole dream feels supernatural, with uncanny feelings and angry ones. But the dream scared and shocked me; it helped me see how I had been neglecting my patient, and I have since been able to correct that."

Survivor Guilt

The therapists who had the "moving picture" dream and the "angry dog" dream were also experiencing survivor guilt, a particularly widespread problem among people who engaged in risky behaviors before HIV was identified, yet somehow managed to survive. Survivor guilt can also be exacerbated by feeling judged by other people. For example, a man whose lover died of AIDS began a new relationship two months after the funeral. He had heard several of his friends speak very contemptuously of people who started new relationships too soon after their lovers had died. And so he was engaged in a complicated deception of keeping his new lover secret from nearly all his friends and family. Since the man was Jewish, I told him that traditional Jewish law requires a mourning period of one year for a parent, but only 30 days for a spouse.[12] The rationale is that one should get on with one's life and not live singly, in suffering, for too long a time. In this way, we could start with a perspective that what he had done had not been sinful in certain cultures, and consider the psychodynamics of those who would condemn him. This detoxified the issue of his guilt, so that eventually we could look into some of the unformulated emotional reactions he had to his lover's death, including suppressed rage, that made him more vulnerable to other people's assessment that he was guilty. And then, we could also look at the characterological issues that were involved in his deceptive way of living.

Survivor guilt, when denied, can lead to various kinds of symptomatology or strange blocks in feeling and behavior. For example, Jack was a perfectionistic, middle-aged gay man who had been in a steady, mostly monogamous relationship with Edward for 23 years and had repeatedly tested HIV-negative. He was proud of this long relationship, but after two years of therapy, he "confessed" to me in one session: "I was able to be there for all my friends who were dying of AIDS except one—that was Louis. I feel so guilty towards him. I didn't spend enough time with him while he was dying of AIDS, and I didn't go to his memorial service. It felt like a compulsion to keep away.

---

12. A rabbi has since told me that my information about the Jewish mourning laws was inaccurate. The actual mourning period may be longer or shorter, depending on whether there are children (Lamm, 1969).

"You see, Louis and I had an on-and-off affair for four years in the 1970s. At one point, I actually was willing to leave Edward for him, but he wasn't interested. He seemed content just to have a sexual liaison with me—with me and many, many other people. The trouble was, I kept contracting minor sexual infections from Louis, like repeated bouts of NSU (nonspecific urethritis). He never showed symptoms, but I did, so I started to feel like his petri dish. I even got to the point where I would take an antibiotic prophylactically before sleeping with him.

"Obviously, this situation could not go on indefinitely, and when he rejected my idea of committing to him, I think the whole thing fell apart, and I decided to stay with Edward. But when AIDS appeared, I got really scared. I just realized (it's amazing—it's taken eight years for me to realize this) that Louis was the one person with whom I had sexual relations where there was a clear and serious risk of my contracting AIDS from him.

"I hadn't heard from him in years, but one day I met him on a train—his leg was extremely swollen from Kaposi's Sarcoma. That is how I found out he had AIDS. Right after I saw him, I went to an isolated place and just started howling. I was so upset—mostly from seeing him suffering so. But wasn't I also weeping for myself, for what could have happened to me, if I hadn't been lucky? Even though I knew I was HIV-negative, seeing him so sick *felt* dangerous to me. It sounds selfish, but I think that's the way it was, and once I admitted this to myself, there was no denying it anymore. Probably, the fact that I *was* trying to deny it is what made my behavior towards him so irrational and bad."

Suicidal Ideation

Another area of change for psychoanalytic thinking has to do with suicidal ideation. Most mental health practitioners have been trained about the dangers of suicidal ideation and its correlation with suicidal attempts and actual suicides. For patients with AIDS, however, I have found that suicidal ideation can sometimes be *helpful.* In an illness in which unpredictability and loss of control are so pronounced, suicidal fantasies give the patient the freedom to fantasize having complete control of his bodily state and his destiny. Paradoxically, the elaboration and exploration of such fantasies within psychotherapy can, in my experience, lessen the likelihood that a patient will actually commit suicide.

For example, I worked with a patient whose health was getting much worse. He spent hours moping or crying in his apartment, and he began to talk to me about suicidal thoughts. We immersed ourselves in talk of death. I asked him how he was thinking about committing suicide. He told me he was thinking of tying a rope around his neck and tying the other end onto something in his apartment. Then he would jump out the window, and be hanging dead outside his building. The fantasy had several important aspects. Other people would be forced to see his misery. He would be relieved of much of the loneliness he felt, even though he would be dead. He would also be making a public statement about his misery and rage about having AIDS and about what he felt was society's relative indifference to AIDS patients. He then told me other fantasies that were even more shocking and destructive, involving public violence. The elaboration and analysis of these fantasies were very helpful to this patient; they brightened his affect, as he felt freer to turn his rage outward rather than inward, and they also led him to see the emotional burden of his isolation, which was partly self-imposed and which he could change.

Some patients who fear suffering and incapacity may stockpile barbiturates or other medications to allow them to commit suicide at some time in the future. In my view, it is contraindicated for a therapist to try to stop such preparations for suicide. We find that, paradoxically, those who take concrete steps to prepare for suicide often do not kill themselves when their physical condition deteriorates. But knowing that they could end things is often very helpful in enabling them to tolerate the pains of the illness. As Shakespeare wrote in *King Lear*, "The worst is not so long as we can say, 'This is the worst'" (IV.i.29–30).

Here, as always, analysis of the countertransference is important. The therapist who has trouble with a patient's suicidal thoughts should ask himself or herself, "What are my own experiences with suicidal thoughts and actions, in others and myself? Have I never had a suicidal thought? What would life be like without the possibility of suicide? Is my reaction against the patient's suicidal thinking possibly fueled by an unconscious *wish* that he commit suicide?" If you can answer these questions honestly, you will be able to work more evenhandedly with your patient's turmoil.

People Having Unsafe Sex and Lying to Their Partners

One of the most troubling situations for the psychotherapist is when a patient who is HIV-positive confides that he is having unsafe sex and lying to his sex partner that he is HIV-negative. The partner's life is thus threatened, and the therapist usually has very strong feelings. One study (Kegeles, Catania, and Coates, 1988) found that 12 percent of individuals undergoing HIV testing would not tell their primary partner if they turned out to be HIV-positive.

There is no easy solution to such a situation. The medicolegal guidelines offer a good deal of latitude (Daniolos and Holmes, 1995) and, in any case, are not an alternative to good clinical judgment. At best, one must steer a course between confronting the patient with the meaning of his action and not alienating him from the therapy. Some therapists feel that such deceptive sexual behavior is tantamount to attempted murder and feel that they must take a strong stand with the patient, at times saying that he must cease such action or terminate the therapy. The risk is that the patient will then feel so judged and threatened that he will stop treatment and continue his behavior anyway.[13] An alternative approach is to try to work with the underlying motives of such a patient. Not infrequently, the patient feels tremendous rage that he has been infected and wishes to infect others who have been more fortunate. At times the rage extends to society's tactless and often cruel treatment of HIV-positive people. In addition, the situation is often not so clear. I have worked with one patient who lied to his sex partners about his HIV status but justified it to himself on the grounds that no one would have sexual relations with him otherwise, and that he was not engaging in any sexual practices that would put his partners at risk for infection, in his opinion. He felt rage at a society that makes the HIV-infected feel like pariahs. Usually such situations require a good deal of work by the psychotherapist on his countertransference, which, if he is HIV-negative, may involve a fantasied identification with the patient's sexual partner. It is useful to consider not only the destructive aspects of the patient's behavior, but the possibly unexpressed needs that it is covering over. Many AIDS patients feel physically shunned and yearn most of all for physical contact, which if it does not involve the exchange of body fluids, is perfectly safe, yet their family and friends may irrationally avoid giving them even a hug.

HIV-Related Issues in HIV-Negative Patients

Another area of psychoanalytic thinking that has been greatly expanded has to do with the pathological consequences of denying, dissociating,

13. See chapter by Dr. Petrucelli for a fine example of the therapist being confronting without being coercive.

and repressing fears of AIDS. The fear of AIDS is having very pervasive effects on the mental health of many patients seen in psychotherapy today; they may be only dimly aware of such fear or too afraid to talk about it with the psychotherapist, let alone with their families and friends. The effect of this unconscious or unacknowledged fear of AIDS may take many clinical forms, including depression, an inability to plan one's life, anxiety attacks, schizoid withdrawal, counterphobic sexual exploits, or psychosomatic symptoms. For example, Lucy was a wealthy, young, beautiful, married woman who was referred to me by a physician because of serious physical symptoms that could not be explained medically. As we developed a trusting psychotherapeutic relationship, Lucy "confessed" that there was one night in which she was extremely angry at her husband, went to a bar, got drunk, and woke up the next morning in a hotel room with a man she did not know. She had no memory of the night's events, but was terrified from then on that she had contracted AIDS. She had never had the HIV-antibody test (by now, several years had passed), and her anxiety only increased.

She asked me how likely it was that she had contracted HIV. I could tell her that it is estimated that the chance of contracting HIV from one act of unprotected heterosexual vaginal intercourse with an infected person is 1 in 500 for a woman, 1 in 700 for a man; from one act of receptive, unprotected anal intercourse with an infected partner, the risk of transmission is 1 in 50 to 100 (Auerbach, Wypijewska, and Brodie, 1994). Often, when patients have engaged in risky behavior and are afraid of contracting AIDS, they ask for such statistics, and it is helpful for the clinician to provide them. But generally, even if the likelihood of transmission is relatively small, the patient's anxiety will not be calmed, and one has to analyze the psychological weight of such statistics.

In the next few sessions, Lucy and I explored her fantasies about AIDS, which were of extreme suffering and were related to religious fantasies of sin and retribution. I eventually told her that I thought her medical symptoms might never resolve without her clarifying the HIV issue. I also told her where and how she could obtain the test privately and confidentially. She had the test, and the result was seronegative. That finding, plus a good deal more psychoanalytic exploration, resolved many of her physical symptoms.

Lucy, like many people, had put her life on hold while ruminating about her fears of AIDS and procrastinating about getting the test. In retrospect, she realized that her unconscious presumption was that she did have AIDS and would die soon, so no major life decisions needed to be made. Usually, people become aware of the *extent* to which they have "put life on hold" only *after* they receive a seronegative test result.

I have seen this phenomenon so often in my practice that I think it might be worth designating it a syndrome—the syndrome of "depression secondary to HIV anxiety." The initial presentation of such patients can be extremely varied, but often, in some way, they seem to be paralyzed. They are going through the motions of life without any clear sense of directing their life course. While there can be many other determinants of such a clinical picture, in the era of AIDS, a major and often unconscious determinant is the fear of having been infected. Such people may not get past their difficulties until they can resolve their terror of being tested. It is important for the clinician to recognize that this syndrome is very pervasive, and not only among the so-called risk groups. It can and does appear in anyone. I have often heard that someone like Lucy, a wealthy married woman, asks her wealthy doctor about AIDS fears, and is told, "Oh, YOU don't need to worry about that." The doctor is involved in a kind of projected denial. He seems to be thinking, "AIDS is not threatening you. Not us. Not me." But anyone who asks about AIDS is worried about it, and if the doctor avoids talking about it or denying the fear, all sorts of psychiatric complications may result.

People like Lucy often want to know how long the incubation period is between HIV infection and the appearance of HIV antibodies on the test. Seroconversion usually occurs within three months, and at most six months. Today, we generally advise patients to have the HIV test three months after the last risk behavior, and then again three months later. Further research may refine or change this procedure. It is also a good idea for patients to obtain the test result immediately before a psychotherapy session. For very anxious patients, the drawing of blood is also best arranged to precede a psychotherapy session.

Dissociated fears of AIDS affect not only patients but their psychotherapists as well. Issues of HIV disease often present themselves even in physically healthy patients, and this stimulates serious questions for the therapist of his own relationship to disease and health, to sexual behavior, drug use, and his own sense of risk of HIV infection. For example, a married female psychoanalytic candidate, in supervision with me, was analyzing a married female patient close to her age. At a certain point, the patient revealed that a number of years before she had been a victim of date-rape with a man that she had since discovered was actively bisexual. She feared that she might have been infected with HIV and yet had not been tested. She had never told her husband, and seemed unconcerned about this. But she presented four dreams in a single session, all of which suggested latent dream thoughts of great fear of being infected, of infecting her husband, and, in the transference, of her therapist being magically able to solve the AIDS danger through great curative powers, perhaps by magically absorbing the disease from her patient. The therapist was notably inactive in this session, making no attempt at interpreting the dreams. In supervision, we discovered that her counterresistance was due to phobic denial, related to the fact that the therapist herself had had some sexual experiences in the past that might have exposed her to HIV, and she had never been tested. The therapist was tested in the next week (she was HIV-negative, fortunately) and was better able from then on to address the patient's fears of contagion, transference fantasies, and resistance to being tested.

Since then, I have seen many psychotherapists in supervision whose work has been constrained, in different ways, by fears of AIDS that have usually not even been acknowledged, let alone worked through. From these experiences, I have come to a principle that applies to every psychotherapist working with AIDS issues, which today is every psychotherapist: *You must have the HIV test yourself.* It is the only way you will gain empathy, not only with your patients' experiences, but with your own unacknowledged fears and illusions. From the moment you make the appointment to have the blood drawn, you will find your mind flooded with special anxieties that are very specific to you. For example, perhaps you feel protected from HIV by the walls of a long-standing monogamous marriage. You may find, during the wait between when the blood is drawn and when you receive the result, that no one is fully confident in a mate's fidelity. You will also realize the stigma and embarrassment—and countless other unpleasant feelings—involved in just going for the test.

HIV Testing and AIDS Anxiety

The test for HIV antibodies has the effect of bringing tremendous anxiety to the fore. Patients who may be at some risk for AIDS can keep their anxiety at bay for years, as long as they are not tested and have no other evidence of the disease. But once the blood for the HIV-antibody test has been drawn, the latent dread emerges. And if, as in some cases, the results will not be available for two or more weeks, the interim time period can be hellish. The defense of denial is suddenly shattered, and the patient is flooded with the real prospect of finding out that he is HIV-positive (Perry et al., 1990). During this time period, it is usually useless to offer reassurances that the patient is relatively unlikely to have been infected with the virus, or that even if infected, illness and death are not necessarily imminent. During such a period, one patient said, "I feel as if someone is holding a gun in front of my forehead, and I know that the bullet in it may be a real one or a blank, and that the trigger will be pulled in two weeks, and there is absolutely nothing I can do about it except worry."

Psychotherapists may be confronted with pathological AIDS anxiety, where a patient develops an intense and persistent fear of AIDS, despite laboratory tests and other evidence that he or she is not infected with HIV. Such patients become extremely vigilant for any physical abnormality, and psychosomatic complaints can at times reach delusional proportions. Although reassurance is not generally useful, a pointed psychoanalytic interpretation can be extremely productive. Often it may be found that other psychological factors, besides real fear of an unknown and unpredictable disease, can be exacerbating the patient's fears.

For example, I treated a single man in his 30s whose primary identifications were split between an extremely aggressive, hypermasculine toughness and a soft, self-abnegating passivity that he identified with women. He was conflicted between a strong sense of guilt and a fascination with violence and crime. This had been clarified by a dream in which he saw the printed message "PRESTYL DOLBY," which he had interpreted as "Press the till, dough'll be yours"; in other words, steal from the cash register. In his fifth year of analysis, he reached a professional milestone for which he had yearned for many years. Almost immediately after this achievement, he noticed some sores in his mouth and a coating on his tongue. He was convinced he had AIDS. He consulted an internist who believed that the symptoms were not serious, but drew blood for an HIV-antibody test. The results would be known in two weeks. The interim period was terrifying for the patient. He continually examined his oral cavity and was convinced that his symptoms were not improving, which he took to be evidence of being immunocompromised. He described canals, ridges, and protrusions around the underside of the tongue. He obtained an ENT consultation, and was diagnosed as having "a normal tongue."

Still the anxiety persisted and even increased. The patient telephoned in a panic. We had an emergency session, during which he reported a dream. "Some people had filled a bathtub with all kinds of groceries, including an open gallon-container of milk. I pissed into the tub, onto the groceries, and even into the open container of milk. I was horrified at what I had done." He felt that the groceries may have been for the religious holidays.

Shortly after telling me the dream, the patient felt an urgent need to urinate, and he wanted to know how much time remained in the session. More than half an hour remained. He said he didn't want to urinate in my bathroom for fear of giving me AIDS. I told him that was not the way AIDS is transmitted. When he returned from the bathroom, I interpreted to him that his comment before going to the bathroom had indicated that he thought of his urine as destructive, to me in fact, and to the "food" in the dream. Although he had felt horrified in the dream about what he had done, he had done it. He then volunteered an important memory. His aunt, an important figure in his life, had once told him that she had stolen money from her father's cash register regularly, in order to collect money for her wedding. I said, "Oh, that was the original prestyl dolby!" (remembering his association, "Press the till, dough'll be yours"). The patient looked confused at first, then sighed and said that the interpretation had felt very strongly affecting; he relaxed and almost fell asleep on the couch. His division of men and women into aggressive criminals and honest nurturers was a defensive distortion that this memory clarified. The patient had a secret pride in his professional achievement and in breaking family conventions, all of which were interacting with issues of gender identity. The fear of AIDS was a fantasied retribution for his guilty thrill at his success.

Just as this patient was irrationally fearful of AIDS, other patients may show an excessive lack of fear of AIDS, but either conscious presentation can conceal the reverse in the unconscious. The psychotherapist needs to be aware that the dread of AIDS can be totally unconscious and may produce unusual symptom pictures that do not appear AIDS-related. One sees very high levels of denial in some patients, and the therapist runs the risk of assuming that something very obvious to him is also noticed by the patient. For example, a gay man in his 30s, John, presented in psychotherapy with severe panic attacks, day and night. During the day he would feel as if he were having a heart attack, and in the middle of the night he would wake up in terror. I asked if he was dreaming when he awoke, and he said that at times he was dreaming that he had AIDS. He was involved in a relationship of two years' standing with a man, Leo. A brief inquiry revealed that Leo's prior lover had died of AIDS, yet Leo had never told John who, three months into the relationship, found out from someone else. John mentioned this discovery to Leo, who had a lame excuse for keeping it secret. John rationalized away his immediate suspicion and then forgot about it (except in his dreams). Leo himself had not been tested for the HIV virus; in fact, he refused to be tested. I commented to John that anyone in a gay relationship today would be concerned about AIDS, and would be especially concerned if his partner had had a long-standing relationship with someone who died of the disease. A person would be further concerned, I said, if the partner had concealed this fact and even more so if the partner had not been tested, especially if the partner *refused* to be tested. John seemed startled by these thoughts; but the anxiety attacks ceased.

HIV Testing and Confidentiality

It is important to recognize that many people do not know how to obtain HIV testing, nor are they secure about the confidentiality. It would be impossible here to catalogue all of the resources for HIV testing. Generally, however, there are several main choices. A county department of health, in many states, will perform the test anonymously and without charge. Such departments often have a relatively long waiting period between the drawing of the blood sample and the reporting of the result, usually one or two weeks. For all patients, this waiting period can be extremely difficult; for some patients it may be intolerable. Private testing facilities can also provide anonymous testing. The patient may make an appointment with them, register under an assumed name, and pay the fee for testing in cash. Patients will, in any case, be given a number that will identify the results without revealing their true name. Some private testing facilities can provide results within 24 hours, which is very much desired by clients who are extremely anxious. A private physician can draw the blood and then submit it anonymously to a testing facility for results. In this case, the identity of the patient will be kept confidential, except to the physician. Some patients prefer this approach, especially if they have a good rapport with their physician. However, if they are very concerned about confidentiality, they should be sure that the physician does not claim the HIV test on insurance forms. The patient can also test his or her own blood, using the home test kit. In this case, a small blood sample is sent to a laboratory, and the result is given over the phone. With this procedure, a patient may find out that he or she is HIV-positive without face-to-face counseling, which poses a certain amount of psychological risk. However, it allows patients who are extremely vigilant about confidentiality to have themselves tested without anyone even seeing them.

I have heard of many other testing procedures. In one rural town, a patient was told that the local medical laboratory could perform the test, but only with prior referral by a physician. The patient felt that confidentiality would be impossible in that situation, and was especially concerned that there was more risk of losing confidentiality in a small town. She chose to go to the county health department, where confidentiality could be assured, even though it meant driving a total of 200 miles for the testing and results. This was before the home test kit was available, which would have obvious benefits in such a case.

The concern about confidentiality may be quite intense; but in our current society, having it known that one is HIV-positive can have serious consequences in one's personal life and career. People have been fired from their jobs, and even if such actions are illegal, the legal action that may be required to set right the injustice may be costly, time consuming, and draining to someone who, being HIV-positive, may not have the resources or the will for such a struggle. Those who discriminate may wager that the patient will die before his legal claims can be won. (The film *Philadelphia* dramatized this situation.)

Public health clinics and many private testing facilities also provide pretest and posttest counseling, which is important. Even if the patient is in psychotherapy, on-site counseling at the moment when someone is informed that he or she is HIV-positive is imperative. Without such counseling, there is the risk that the patient, hearing of the seropositive result, may commit suicide. I often arrange with patients to obtain the test result immediately before a psychotherapy session with me. Often the drawing of blood is also best arranged to precede the psychotherapy session.

The terror of AIDS can be exacerbated by a number of unconscious fears. One man I worked with had a fairly marginal risk of infection, but he was unusually terrified by death, having seen one of his parents die before his eyes when he was a child. He was planning to be married and felt he had to have an HIV test before the wedding, but he could not bring himself to do so. Finally, he needed to change insurance plans, and so he applied for a policy that he knew screened applicants for HIV. He presumed that if he was given the insurance policy, he would be uninfected. He was given the policy, but even then he could not bring himself to ask the examining physician for the results of the HIV test.

Unconscious Factors in Assessing One's Risk for HIV

The assessment of one's risk for HIV is highly subjective and can be influenced by many unconscious factors, which can include the sense of immortality in the young, as well as masochistic and suicidal tendencies. Just as there can be pathologically excessive fear of AIDS, there can also be manifestly inadequate fear of AIDS, and this can become the subject of psychotherapeutic inquiry. For example, a gay man in his 20s came to me for analysis. He had been depressed since he was a child, and I noted that he often engaged in "privately suicidal actions"; they did not draw public attention, but people who knew him well could certainly have seen that they were self-destructive. His parents were educated and apparently concerned with their children, but were also quite self-involved and unreliable. When the patient was seven years old, he climbed onto the roof of his house during a thunderstorm and began cleaning the leaves from the gutter. This was dangerous in many ways: the roof was three stories above ground, it was slippery from the rain, and there was danger of electrocution from the lightning, but his parents took no notice. In our work together, "going up on the roof" became a metaphor for risking one's life.

After one of my vacations, he reported that he had met a man with whom he had a brief sexual liaison. When they got into bed, he felt swollen lymph nodes in the other man's back, but proceeded anyway. I interpreted that such an action was suicidal, that "he had gone up on the roof" during my absence. He claimed that I was being an alarmist. (This was in 1983, when public awareness of AIDS was not as great as today, but there was enough information available for me to be greatly concerned.) Several years later, he no longer considered me an alarmist, claiming instead that my alarm may have saved his life, and he realized how he had integrated the AIDS risk into his privately suicidal behavior.

When there have been long-standing suicidal or self-destructive trends, a patient may incorporate AIDS into this personality structure. For example, I worked with a heterosexual young man who was unconsciously suicidal for much of his life. He told me that he had been sleeping with a lot of women on one-night stands without a condom, risking AIDS and getting someone pregnant. When I asked him if he did other suicidal things, he seemed startled that I called his sexual experiences "suicidal." But then he told me of a dream he had had four times.

"I am in a bar, a house or somewhere. I am sitting at a table with one or two people and I have one or two beers. All of a sudden, I put my face down on the table, and I couldn't move. I couldn't move. I am screaming to the others, 'Wait, I'm coming!' but I have no control over anything."

I noted that one meaning of the dream is that he is ruining his body and that others don't notice. He then told me about his extensive drug and steroid use. He had a kind of double consciousness, of denial and panic at the same time. In the dream, the sign of his liveliness is his screaming, "I'm coming," his sexual ejaculation, but it is an empty, panicky signal amidst a total paralysis and loss of control.

Cultural Determinants in AIDS Issues

The assessment of pathologically excessive fear of AIDS and inadequate fear of AIDS often makes the psychotherapist keenly aware of cultural differences. Many IV drug users do not share the middle-class view of what is appropriate fear. If one has grown up in severe poverty and faced a high risk of death from street crime, hunger, and disease, and if one's hopes for betterment are slim, then the threat of AIDS as a killer does not loom so large in the universe of dangers.

"When you tell black South Africans, 'Here's a disease that will kill you young, keep you from getting work and make you discriminated against,' that's nothing new to them," said Mary Crewe, who runs the Community AIDS Center in Johannesburg. "Your chances of being killed in a train attack, or fighting in the townships, or in a police crossfire, are probably greater than contracting the virus. If you say to people who are HIV-positive, 'Reduce stress, eat well and get enough sleep,' if you are a black South African at the moment, it is very difficult to do any of those things." The same may be true for many Americans who live in the inner cities or in other impoverished circumstances.

For an HIV-positive woman whose culture deems that motherhood is the raison d'être of a woman's life, the warning that without medication there is a one-third chance that her baby will be HIV-positive and die of AIDS may not deter her at all. More than one such would-be mother has replied, "One in three? That's not so bad. I've got a two-out-of-three chance that the baby won't get sick."

In 1994, it was found that if a mother was treated with AZT, the chances of her transmitting the virus to her child were reduced from 26 percent to 8 percent (Connor et al., 1994). But it was also found that damage to heart function occurred in many newborn children exposed to AZT in utero (Domanski et al., 1995). Since then, it has also been found that the higher the viral load of the mother, the more likely is transmission of the virus to the fetus (Dickover et al., 1996), and because most of the transmission of HIV to the infant occurs during delivery, a delivery by cesarean section reduces the chance of infection of the infant (European Collaborative Study, 1994). In view of these findings, if an HIV-positive woman chooses to become pregnant, there are many practical choices for her to make, and the psychotherapist may help the patient sort through the latest research findings.

Negotiating Safer Sex in an Unsafe World

Until there is a cure for AIDS, the greatest hope for limiting the disease is by preventing its transmission. But the most powerful tool for doing so is not a preachy, scientific account of the facts of HIV transmission. It is a common finding that heterosexual college students can recite accurately all the ways that AIDS is transmitted and all the ways that AIDS can be prevented but simultaneously do not follow those rules.

Falling in love is a kind of "normal abnormality." We develop all sorts of exaggerated notions about the goodness of the beloved. The wish to idealize the loved one does not fit with the notion of fearing contagion. Those who try to educate the young about AIDS and its transmission need to recognize the sorts of irrational ideas that pervade romantic idealization and lead to undue risk-taking. These ideas include:

1. As long as I am not gay or an IV drug user, I am safe from HIV.
2. I can tell by looking at someone if he or she is HIV-positive.
3. If he (or she) really loves me, of course he (or she) would not give me HIV.[14]
4. I am immortal and will live forever.

The last notion is a very common idea of adolescence. One would almost say it is a normal irrational idea, connected in part with the feeling of great adventure among adolescents and the sense of infinite possibility.

Adolescence is the time when we consider what we are going to do with our lives; we revel in the joy of anticipating the future, of the heady choice between different alternatives in careers, mates, and love. Part of the experience of adolescence is sexual experimentation. In our culture, a certain amount of dating and sexual play, in order to gain social and romantic experience, is thought to be a good thing.

Ultimately, the most powerful instigator to behavior change is confrontation with someone who has contracted HIV and who is in a very similar life situation. One of the most powerful defenses against safer sex is the belief that AIDS happens to other people. Another barrier to safer sex is the common adolescent attitude, "Who cares? Life is full of dangers." In my view, the film *KIDS*[15] should be required viewing for all teenagers. It tells the story of a boy who is obsessed with deflowering virgins. One of the girls, who has had only one sexual experience with him, finds out that he has given her HIV, and spends the rest of the movie looking for him in order to tell him. It gets across to teenagers the reality of HIV infection in a context that is very real to teenage life and sexuality in our era.

---

14. Sometimes it is transmitted without the infected person's knowledge that he is HIV-positive (e.g., *The New York Times*, July 26, 1996).

15. Incidentally, the logo for the movie *KIDS* subtly mirrors the logo for AIDS, and makes clear that there is only one letter different between the two.

Teaching young people the facts about AIDS is essential, but it is important to recognize that when a subject is as fraught with anxiety as AIDS is, people may jump to wrong conclusions or misunderstand the facts as we know them. Washington (1995) has provided a searing first-person account of a young man's psychology while engaging in unsafe sex. When the young man learned that experts thought a 10 percent bleach solution killed the AIDS virus in needles, he started to give himself a bleach enema after having anal sex. Not only would that not protect against HIV, the internal trauma caused by the bleach might actually have increased his risk of infection.

Even those who know the facts about HIV transmission may find it difficult to implement that knowledge in the actual experience of dating and lovemaking. For example, some men balk at the use of condoms and are insulted when their female partners insist on them (Amaro, 1995). They may feel that the demand for a condom implies that they are gay and may then insist on unprotected sex in order to "prove their masculinity." In addition, many men may find condoms physically distasteful or may find themselves too carried away by passion to interrupt it with putting on a condom (Davies, 1993; Ehrhardt, Yingling, and Warne, 1991).

Finding a comfortable, relatively consistent basis of behavior is necessary for every person who is sexually active and not in a securely monogamous relationship. One can identify two polarities of approach to HIV infection and risk reduction—the maximally avoidant and the maximally permissive. The epitome of the maximally avoidant approach is abstinence. This is the approach for unmarried people that is favored by certain religious organizations, such as the Catholic Church, and it has been adopted by certain people out of their own convictions or fears. The biggest risk of abstinence is that there will be lapses in abstinence, what in alcoholism is called "falling off the wagon." Sexuality is such a powerful force in human living, and such a major source of the joy in living, that to give it up entirely is a serious task, and probably not realistic for most people. Masturbation is totally safe from an HIV standpoint, but it is not satisfactory to many people as a sexual outlet because it lacks the intimacy and sensual excitement of another person, and it is lonely.

I would not dissuade someone from abstinence who has chosen it, feels comfortable with it, and can achieve it. If it means, however, that someone will be mostly abstinent, but will then have episodes of dissociated, unsafe sexual contact, that is a very serious and dangerous situation. In other words, abstinence is fine for those who can maintain it—but few can. This was well dramatized in the film and play *Jeffrey*. Saint Paul also noted the individual differences in capacity for abstinence when he said, "It is better to marry than to burn" (I Cor. 7:9).

If a single person who is not in a monogamous relationship does not choose abstinence, he or she must face the difficult question of which sexual acts to engage in and how. Within the gay community, there has been much debate on this subject. On the side of greater permissiveness, Walter Odets (1995; Senterfitt, 1995) has argued that exaggerating the risk of too many sexual behaviors that he considers not very risky may lead many gay men to totally abandon any attempt at protecting themselves. He has argued that the risk of infection through oral sex is minimal and, therefore, gay men should be told that the main precaution they need to use is a condom during anal sex. If they are in an ongoing, monogamous relationship with someone who is HIV-negative, they can even dispense with condoms.

But there are other reports of HIV being transmitted through oral sex (e.g., Lifson et al., 1990; Samuel et al., 1993; Rotello, 1994; Baba et al., 1994), albeit less frequently and less efficiently than through vaginal or anal intercourse. The choice of what to consider an acceptable level of risk must be a personal decision (Johnston, 1995), but when the psychotherapist and the patient have different views on the subject, it can be a difficult area for discussion. Certainly, if a patient is engaging in clearly unsafe sex (e.g., receptive anal intercourse without a condom), the psychotherapist should not mince words that this is dangerous behavior.

I once saw a psychotherapist in supervisory consultation who was an adherent of self psychology. He was working with a patient who had been repeatedly engaging in clearly unsafe sex. But since the therapist's credo of working was to immerse himself in the patient's subjective viewpoint, he only "mirrored" the patient's view that his behavior was harmless. When his patient seroconverted, he felt extremely guilty, and both he and the patient regretted their acceptance of the behavior.[16]

People having relatively unsafe sex may often speak self-righteously and with bravado about feeling comfortable with what they are doing. In such instances, their dreams may show the other side of their feelings, which can include much more fright and self-doubt. For example, I worked in psychoanalysis with a man in his mid-30s who had an affair with an HIV-positive man. They had abided by safer-sex guidelines with regard to anal intercourse, but not for oral sex. He dismissed any questions I had about the safety of what he was doing. After the relationship ended, his self-confidence withered. He feared being tested for HIV and used many rationalizations to avoid it. Then he brought in the following dream.

"I'm in a very nice neighborhood. There are wide streets and big

16. See the chapters by Petrucelli and Mujica for further discussions of this issue.

houses, like in Garden City or Deal, NJ. It is during the daytime. It's cloudy. I'm with my friend Maria. We are walking down the sidewalk, walking and talking. Then we were in someone's backyard. It was behind someone's white garage. On the side of the garage were two snakes. They were fairly big. I was wondering, were they dangerous or not? One was orange and black. It looked like a rattlesnake."

The patient mentioned that he had recently read an article about snakes taking over Fiji. They bite babies. Then he asked me, "What do snakes mean in dreams? Don't they mean penises?" He then went on to connect the two penises in his dream to the two penises in his sexual life, and the question about whether his behavior had been dangerous. Maria represented not only his friend, but the Virgin Mary, who would not get into such a predicament, and from whom the patient hoped to receive religious salvation. He said, "I've been thinking about getting retested, just to put closure on that period of my life. Maybe after the New Year."

AIDS and Syphilis

When AIDS first appeared we were shocked by it; it was frightening, destructive, and mysterious. It seemed terrifying and without precedent. But as time has passed, and some of the mystery has lessened, we can see that it is a sexually transmitted disease that is, in many ways, similar to syphilis, despite certain medical and biological differences. They are both involved with sex and blood products, either of which can transmit them. Both may have a long incubation period, during which the illness is mostly innocuous or invisible, except through laboratory test. With syphilis, three stages are identified: primary, secondary, tertiary. AIDS has also been divided into three stages: HIV infection, AIDS-related complex (ARC), and "full-blown" AIDS (although the use of the ARC diagnosis has receded over the years).

Both AIDS and syphilis have occurred most frequently in young people, and have made death in the third and fourth decade of life common. They both eventually can affect many different bodily systems and can cause blindness. Syphilis, in its time, was called "the great pretender," because it was often misdiagnosed as other physiological ailments that it mimicked. Similarly, in the early days of AIDS, people were often thought to have just one of the illnesses that were typical, like shingles, thrush, or lymphoma. In fact, during at least the first decade of AIDS, most women who had AIDS were misdiagnosed as having some infection or cancer of the reproductive organs, without recognizing the source of that illness in HIV. Many women died of AIDS without ever being diagnosed as having AIDS.

Both AIDS and syphilis took on significant symbolic meanings in our culture, such as sexual sin and poverty (see Sontag, 1989). Both were spread throughout the world by long-distance travel, to areas that had been completely uninfected. In the case of AIDS, however, transmission has been much faster, thanks to modern advances in travel. Sherwin Nuland (1993) has called AIDS a "jet-propelled disease."

Syphilis was often attributed to the other or the foreigner, much like AIDS (Henig, 1995). The Germans called syphilis "the French disease," the French called it "the Neapolitan disease," the Dutch called it "the Spanish disease," and the Japanese called it "the Chinese ulcer."

There used to be special journals devoted to syphilology, just as today there are special journals devoted to AIDS research and treatment. And both AIDS and syphilis became entrenched parts of the culture and the arts. Both are portrayed as having drastic, profound effects on social and psychic life. An excellent example is Ibsen's *The Wild Duck,* which deals very much with illusion and truth-telling. The play is about unspoken secrets that affect people's lives, and one of those secrets is syphilis. Throughout the play, there is the shadow of the father's syphilis, which is probably responsible for his daughter's vision difficulties.

Today, we see AIDS becoming an increasingly pervasive presence in virtually every art form, including film (*Longtime Companion, Forrest Gump, Trainspotting*), theater (*The Normal Heart, Jeffrey*), music (Corigliano's Symphony No. 1), photography and painting (examplified by Robert Mapplethorpe, Keith Haring, David Wojnarowicz), literature (*A Home at the End of the World, Borrowed Time*), poetry (see Klein, 1989), and dance (works by Bill T. Jones). At the same time, AIDS has depleted the ranks of the great artists of our time, just as syphilis did in previous centuries.

Both AIDS and syphilis can directly cause psychiatric and neurological problems. The spirochete that causes syphilis, *treponema pallidum,* can attack the nervous system directly, as can HIV. Before penicillin, a very common psychiatric diagnosis was "syphilis-caused psychosis." In 1940, 6.1 per 100,000 first admissions to a psychiatric hospital were for tertiary syphilis. And HIV can similarly cause cognitive deficits, perhaps quite subtly in the early years of infection, and may later cause more severe psychiatric symptoms of psychosis or dementia (Atkinson and Grant, 1994).

The close link between HIV and neuropsychiatric functioning is one of the reasons that AIDS has received more attention than most other serious medical illnesses by the mental health community. Another reason is that AIDS is very much connected with sexual behavior, and sexuality has often been closely connected with emotional experience, psychiatry, and psychoanalysis. Here, there is another parallel between AIDS and syphilis. At the turn of the century, Sigmund Freud noted that many of the neurotic patients that he saw had syphilis in their own or their parents' history.

Freud thought that syphilis played a pivotal role in the psychopathology of many of the cases he saw, a fact that was ignored or denied by many medical authorities. In a footnote to the Dora case, for example, he wrote (1905):

> to my mind, however, there is another factor which is of more significance in the girl's hereditary or, properly speaking, constitutional predisposition. I have mentioned that her father had contracted syphilis before his marriage. Now a *strikingly high* percentage of the patients whom I have treated psychoanalytically come of fathers who have suffered from tabes or general paralysis. . . . Syphilis in the male parent is a very relevant factor in the aetiology of the neuropathic constitution of children [pp. 20–21n].

Thus, the kinds of interaction between AIDS and psychopathology that we see today are not as new as many people think. There were similar interconnections between syphilis and psychopathology in Freud's day. The syphilis spirochete affected the brain and nervous system, causing psychiatric symptoms; the investigation of syphilitic histories often uncovered secrets and marital complications that clarified the psychodynamics of parents and the psychological development of children within the family; and all of these factors heightened the significance of sexuality in psychiatry. When a cure for AIDS is discovered, we must guard against presuming that there will be no serious new sexually transmitted diseases in the future, and that the interaction between sexually transmitted disease and psychiatry no longer requires our attention. In some form, it will probably be a fact of life for all future generations.

After the Cure

As I was preparing this book, I noticed that I was having a recurrent fantasy. What if a cure for AIDS is discovered before it is published? How will all of these observations and discoveries change? Will any of them matter? I think this fantasy has many functions, but it is primarily a wish. The wish and the hope that this nightmare called AIDS will end keeps me from burning out. And when it does end, we will all have learned some important lessons.

The Illusion of Man's Ability to Conquer Disease

We will have learned that modern medicine is not omnipotent, and that nature will always have some new tricks up her sleeve. It took mankind about 400 years between first identifying syphilis as a disease and finding a cure. During that time, syphilis killed millions. Compare those 400 years with the approximately 40 years between the discovery of penicillin and the appearance of AIDS, and you realize it was just a brief instant that modern man could enjoy the illusion that there were no incurable sexually transmitted diseases and that there would be no more. Although sexual freedom seems quite entrenched in our culture, we can work to integrate it with prudence regarding sexual activities with multiple partners. It would be good to remember that, even when a cure for AIDS is found, other sexually transmitted diseases may well be incubating. Sexual intercourse is an especially efficient route for transmitting microorganisms of all kinds, and anyone choosing to have multiple partners should seriously consider using condoms as a barrier to transmission of whatever possible microorganisms there might be. It is a sad lesson of the AIDS epidemic that many of those who died of the disease had no idea that AIDS existed at the time that they were infected. The lengthy incubation period of this illness could be characteristic of other illnesses whose existence we do not yet know about.

The Need for Social Changes

AIDS has reminded us of the crucial role that social policy can play in shaping psychological experience and human behavior. The morals, inhibitions, and taboos of our society have seriously shaped the spread of AIDS. Our society marginalizes and condemns intravenous drug users, yet we do not supply adequate programs for detoxification. An IV drug user who wants to avoid AIDS frequently finds that there is a long waiting list to get into a detox program, and that in the meantime, there is a social policy that is at odds with providing him or her with clean needles. A society that condemns certain kinds of behavior without providing optimal conditions to favor other kinds of behavior is cruel and self-defeating.

A similar contradictory pattern has exacerbated the AIDS epidemic among gay men, who were the first group to get AIDS in our culture. Society has created an impossible double bind for gay men, on one hand condemning their purported promiscuity, and on the other hand denying them the social institution that is most effective in our culture in limiting promiscuity—marriage. A proportion of gay men managed to stay in monogamous relationships in any case, and they may have been protected from AIDS in that way. During the epidemic, many additional gay men found that monogamous relationships, once thought to be oppressive and confining, became the path to greater sexual excitement and fulfillment. If two people who are both HIV-negative can trust one another to be faithful, then any sexual act between them is safe.

Maintaining such a monogamous relationship, however, is made difficult in our society. If you are heterosexual and married, you know that sustaining a monogamous and fulfilling marriage is not an easy thing. It takes work and imagination. But consider, however hard it is for you to make your marriage work, what would your marriage be like if, as occurs with gay people, public knowledge of your relationship could lead to your losing your job? What if you had to act at work as if your husband or wife didn't exist? What if you had to always say "I" when you meant "we"? What if, in addition, large segments of the population declared in public speeches that your wish to sustain your monogamous relationship publicly and to obtain legal recognition of it was sinful and evil? No doubt, your marriage would be less likely to survive (Blechner, 1995b).

There is no substitute for the legal and economic sanctions of marriage to structure sexuality and foster long-term commitments. If society is truly interested in limiting the spread of the AIDS epidemic and in limiting future epidemics of sexually transmitted diseases, it will take further steps to legitimize gay marriage, to reward and affirm the pledge made by any two individuals, heterosexual or homosexual, to commit themselves to care for each other, to love one another, and to remain faithful to one another.

Value of Psychotherapy for Other Serious Physical Illnesses

We will also have learned the value of psychotherapy for people with serious physical illnesses to improve their quality of life, to enhance their use of medical resources, to ameliorate the course of the illness, and, perhaps, to extend longevity. Virtually everything that I have mentioned concerning the experience of AIDS—the value of certain defenses, the reassessment of one's life, the potential for character change under pressure, the adaptive use of suicidal ideation, the balance of hope and despair, the clarifying value of dreams, the problem of loneliness, and the process of bereavement—applies to people who have life-threatening illnesses other than AIDS. Whether psychotherapy services will be made available to people with other illnesses remains to be seen. Green (1989) has argued that the production of such services on a large scale requires activism within the patient population, and perhaps an identification with the patient group among psychological caregivers.

I recently spoke to a man who had just been diagnosed with prostate cancer. He was looking for a therapy group where he could discuss his emotional experience and was having a very hard time finding one. Why did prostate cancer receive so little attention from psychotherapists? It is possible that many people consider serious illness to be something that should not be spoken about openly. Older friends have told me that early in the 20th century one simply did not use the word "cancer" in polite conversation. At most, one could say "a long illness." Death itself was subject to a similar taboo. Kübler-Ross has worked to dispel this taboo, but it is only somewhat attenuated.

In addition, it seems that most illnesses for which silence has been broken are those that affect groups that are in some way stigmatized by society. We have already seen this to be the case with the gay men and IV drug users who have been the first to get AIDS in the United States. Interestingly, the cancer victims who have mobilized most effectively for better medical and mental health care are those with breast cancer, which affects women predominantly. Breast-cancer activist groups have learned many lessons from the experiences of AIDS activists. By contrast, prostate cancer affects men, and men in general suffer the least prejudice in our society. Also, because men are raised in most societies not to complain, it is not so surprising that they would be less likely to demand mental health services for those with prostate cancer. If such stereotyping were identified and worked through, mental health services could become more readily available to people with all kinds of serious illness. We hope that the knowledge gained from working with people with AIDS, as presented in this book, will be useful to those with other serious illnesses.

References

Abrams, D. (1990), Alternative therapies in HIV infection. *AIDS,* 4:1179–1187.

——— (1992), Dealing with alternative therapies for HIV. In: *The Medical Management of AIDS,* ed. M. Sande & P. Volberding. Philadelphia: Saunders, pp. 111–128.

Adler, G., Beiser, M., Cole, R., Johnston, L. & Krant, M. (1975), Approaches to intervention with dying patients and their families: A case discussion. In: *Bereavement,* ed. B. Schoenberg, I. Gerber, A. Wiener, A. Kutscher, D. Peretz & A. Carr. New York: Columbia

University Press, pp. 281–293.

Amaro, H. (1995), Love, sex, and power: Considering women's realities in HIV prevention. *Amer. Psychol.*, 50:437–447.

Atkinson, J. H. & Grant, I. (1994), Natural history of neuropsychiatric manifestations of HIV disease. *Psychiatr. Clinics N. Amer.*, 17:17–31.

Auerbach, J., Wypijewska, C. & Brodie, H., eds. (1994), *AIDS and Behavior.* Washington, DC: National Academy Press.

Baba, T., Koch, J., Mittler, E., Greene, M., Wyand, M., Penninck, D. & Ruprecht, R. (1994), Mucosal infection of neonatal rhesus monkeys with cell-free SIV. *AIDS Res. & Human Retroviruses*, 10:351–357.

Bayer, P. (1989), A life in limbo. *New York Times Magazine*, April 2.

Blechner, M. J. (1986), Transmission of AIDS from female to male. Letter to *The New York Times*, July 31.

——— (1992), Working in the countertransference. *Psychoanal. Dial.*, 2:161–179.

——— (1993), Psychoanalysis and HIV disease. *Contemp. Psychoanal.*, 29:61–80.

——— (1995a), Schizophrenia. In: *Handbook of Interpersonal Psychoanalysis*, ed. M. Lionells, J. Fiscalini, C. Mann & D. Stern. Hillsdale, NJ: The Analytic Press, pp. 375–396.

——— (1995b), The shaping of psychoanalytic theory and practice by cultural and personal biases about sexuality. In: *Disorienting Sexuality*, ed. T. Domenici & R. Lesser. New York: Routledge, pp. 265–288.

——— (1996), Comments on the theory and therapy of borderline personality disorder. *Contemp. Psychoanal.*, 32:68–73.

Boccaccio, G. (1353), *The Decameron*, trans. G. McWilliam. New York: Penguin, 1972.

Buchbinder, S., Mann, D., Louie, L., Villinger, F., Katz, M. & Holmberg. S. (1993), Healthy long-term positives (HLPs): Genetic cofactors for delayed HIV disease progression. *Abstract of the 9th International Conference on AIDS* (Abstract No. WS-B03-2), Berlin.

Callen, M. (1991), *Surviving AIDS.* New York: HarperCollins.

Cao, Y., Qin, L., Zhang, L., Safrit, J. & Ho, D. (1995), Virologic and immunologic characteristics of long-term survivors of human immunodeficiency virus type 1 infection. *New Engl. J. Med.*, 332:201–207.

Connor, E., Sperling, R. Gelber, R., Kiselev, P., Scott, G., O'Sullivan, M., Van Dyke, R. & Bey, M. (1994), Reduction of maternal-infant transmission of human immunodeficiency virus type 1 with AZT treatment. *New Engl. J. Med.*, 331:1222–1225.

Daniolos, P. & Holmes, V. (1995), HIV public policy and psychiatry: An examination of ethical issues and professional guidelines.

Psychosoma., 36:12–21.

Dansky, S. (1994), *Now Dare Everything.* New York: Harrington Park Press.

Davies, P. (1993), Perspectives on fucking. In: *Sex, Gay Men, and AIDS.* London: Falmer Press, pp. 127–146.

Dickover, R., Garraty, E., Herman, S., Sim, M., Plaeger, S., Boyer, P., Keller, M., Deveikis, A., Stiehm, E. & Bryson, Y. (1996), Identification of levels of maternal HIV-1 RNA associated with risk of perinatal transmission: Effect of maternal Zidovudine treatment on viral load. *J. Amer. Med. Assn.*, 275:599–605.

Domanski, M., Sloase, M., Follmann, D., Scalise, P., Tucker, E., Egan, D. & Pizzo, P. (1995), Effect of AZT and didanosine treatment on heart function in children infected with human immunodeficiency virus. *J. Pediat.*, 127:137–146.

Domarus, E. von (1944), The specific laws of logic in schizophrenia. In: *Language and Thought in Schizophrenia,* ed. J. S. Kasanin. New York: Norton, pp. 104–114.

Ehrhardt, A., Yingling, S. & Warne, P. (1991), Sexual behavior in the era of AIDS: What has changed in the United States? *Annu. Rev. Sex Research,* 2:25–47.

Eissler, K. (1955), *The Psychiatrist and the Dying Patient.* New York: International Universities Press.

European Collaborative Study (1994), Cesarean section and risk of vertical transmission of HIV-1 infection. *Lancet,* 343:1464–1467.

Fawzy, F., Fawzy, N., Hyun, C., Elashoff, R., Guthrie, D., Fahey, J. & Morton, D. (1993), Malignant melanoma: Effects of an early structured psychiatric intervention, coping, and affective state on recurrence and survival 6 years later. *Arch. Gen. Psychiat.*, 50:681–689.

Ferenczi, S. & Rank, O. (1923), *The Development of Psycho-Analysis.* New York: Dover, 1956.

Freud, S. (1900) The interpretation of dreams. *Standard Edition,* 4 & 5. London: Hogarth Press, 1953.

——— (1901), The psychopathology of everyday life. *Standard Edition,* 6. London: Hogarth Press, 1960.

——— (1905), Fragment of an analysis of a case of hysteria. *Standard Edition,* 7:7–122. London: Hogarth Press, 1953.

——— (1917), Mourning and melancholia. *Standard Edition,* 14:243–258. London: Hogarth Press, 1957.

——— (1918), From the history of an infantile neurosis. *Standard Edition,* 17:7–122. London: Hogarth Press, 1955.

——— (1937), Analysis terminable and interminable. *Standard Edition,* 23:216–253. London: Hogarth Press, 1964.

Gerber, M. (1995), *Vice Versa.* New York: Simon and Schuster.

Goldman, S. (1989), Bearing the unbearable: The psychological impact of AIDS. In: *Gender in Transition,* ed. J. Offerman-Zuckerberg. New York: Plenum, pp. 263–274.

Graves, R. (1955), *The Greek Myths.* London: Penguin.

Green, J. (1989), Counselling for HIV infection and AIDS: The past and the future. *AIDS Care,* 1:5–11.

Greenberg, J. (1994), An alternative treatment activist manifesto. *GMHC Treatment Issues,* 7:1–2.

Hausman, K. (1993), Needle-exchange programs effective but controversial. *Psychiat. News,* Sept. 3:11.

Henig, R. M. (1995), The lessons of syphilis in the age of AIDS. *Civilization,* 2:36–43.

Herek, G. & Capitanio, J. (1993), Public reaction to AIDS in the United States: A second decade of stigma. *Amer. J. Public Health,* 83:574–577.

HIV Center for Clinical and Behavioral Studies Report (1991), New York State Psychiatric Institute, Vol. 1, May.

Johnston, W. (1995), *HIV-Negative.* New York: Plenum.

Karel, R. (1993), Needle-exchange program yielding great success. *Psychiat. News,* Jan. 1:10–11.

Kegeles, S., Catania, J. & Coates, T. (1988), Intentions to communicate positive HIV-antibody status to sex partners. *J. Amer. Med. Assn.,* 259: 216–217.

Kernberg, O. (1980), *Internal World and External Reality.* New York: Jason Aronson.

King, P. (1980), The life cycle as indicated by the nature of the transference in the psychoanalysis of the middle-aged and the elderly. *Internat. J. Psycho-anal.,* 61:153–160.

Klein, M. (1989), *Poets for Life.* New York: Crown.

Kübler-Ross, E. (1969), *On Death and Dying.* New York: Macmillan.

——— (1987), *AIDS: The Ultimate Challenge.* New York: Macmillan.

Lamm, M. (1969), *The Jewish Way in Death and Mourning.* Middle Village, NY: Jonathan David Publishers.

Lifson, A., O'Malley, P., Hessol, N., Buchbinder, S., Cannon, L. & Rutherford, G. (1990), HIV seroconversion in two homosexual men after receptive oral intercourse with ejaculation: Implications for counseling concerning safe sexual practices. *Amer. J. Pub. Health,* 80:1509–1511.

Marris, P. (1958), *Widows and Their Families.* London: Routledge & Kegan Paul.

Maslow, A. (1967), Neurosis as a failure of personal growth. *Humanitas,* 3:153–169.

McCutchan, J. (1994), Unproven and unconventional therapies. In: *Textbook of AIDS Medicine,* ed. S. Broder, T. Merigan & D. Bolognesi.

Baltimore: Williams & Wilkins, pp. 807–812.

Mellors, J., Rinaldo, C., Gupta, P., White, R., Todd, J. & Kingsley, L. (1996), Prognosis in HIV-1 infection predicted by the quantity of virus in plasma. *Science,* 272:1167–1170.

Monette, P. (1994), *Last Watch of the Night.* New York: Harcourt Brace.

Myers, W. (1987), Age, rage, and the fear of AIDS. *J. Geriat. Psychiat.,* 20:125–140.

Nuland, S. B. (1993), *How We Die.* New York: Knopf.

Odets, W. (1995), *In the Shadow of the Epidemic.* Durham, NC: Duke University Press.

Osborn, J. (1992), Interview with June Osborn. *The Advocate,* Sept. 8:40–43.

Pantaleo, G., Menzo, S., Vaccarezza, M., Graniosi, C., Cohen, O., Demarest, B., Montefiori, D., Orenstein, J., Gox, C., Schrager, L., Margolick, J., Buchbinder, S., Giorgi, J. & Fauci, A. (1995), Studies in subjects with long-term nonprogressive human immunodeficiency virus infection. *New Engl. J. Med.,* 332:209–216.

Perry, S. W., Jacobsberg, L., Fishman, B., Weiler, P., Gold, J. & Frances, A. (1990), Psychological responses to serological testing for HIV. *AIDS,* 4: 145–152.

Rees, W. D. (1975), The bereaved and their hallucinations. In: *Bereavement,* ed. B. Schoenberg, I. Gerber, A. Wiener, A. Kutscher, D. Peretz, & A. Carr. New York: Columbia University Press.

Rotello, G. (1994), Watch your mouth. *Out,* June:148–168.

Rowland, C. (1988), A view from the moon: A message from one person with AIDS. In: *The Sourcebook on Lesbian/Gay Health Care,* ed. M. Shernoff & W. Scott. Washington, DC: National Lesbian/Gay Health Foundation, pp. 183–186.

Samuel, M., Hessol, N., Shiboski, S., Engel, R., Speed, T. & Winkelstein, W. (1993), Factors associated with human immunodeficiency virus seroconversion in homosexual men in three San Francisco cohort studies, 1984–1989. *J. Acquired Immunodeficiency Syndrome,* 6:303–312.

Schaffner, B. (1990), Reactions of medical personnel and intimates to persons with AIDS. In: *Behavioral Aspects of AIDS,* ed. D. Ostrow. New York: Plenum Press, pp. 341–354.

——— (1994), The crucial and difficult role of the psychotherapist in the treatment of the HIV-positive patient. *J. Amer. Acad. Psychoanal.,* 22:505–518.

Schwartzberg, S. (1993), Struggling for meaning: How HIV-positive gay men make sense of AIDS. *Profess. Psychol.: Research & Practice,* 24:483–490.

——— (1994), Vitality and growth in HIV-infected gay men. *Soc. Sci.*

Med., 38:593–602.

Sechehaye, M. (1951), *Symbolic Realization.* New York: International Universities Press.

Senterfitt, W. (1995), HIV prevention for gay men. *Being Alive Newsletter,* Aug., p. 1.

Shenon, P. (1996), AIDS epidemic, late to arrive, now explodes in populous Asia. *New York Times,* Jan. 21, pp. 1, 8.

Shernoff, M. (1991), Eight years of working with people with HIV: The impact upon a therapist. In: *Gays, Lesbians, and Their Therapists,* ed. C. Silverstein. New York: Norton, pp. 227–239.

Shilts, R. (1987), *And the Band Played On. New York: St. Martin's Press.*

Sontag, S. (1989), *AIDS and Its Metaphors.* New York: Farrar, Straus & Giroux.

Spiegel, D., Bloom, J., Kraemer, H. & Gottheil, E. (1989), Effect of psychosocial treatment on survival of patients with metastatic breast cancer. *Lancet,* 2:888–891.

Sullivan, H. S. (1924), Schizophrenia: Its conservative and malignant features. In: *Schizophrenia as a Human Process.* New York: Norton, 1962.

Szalita, A. (1974), Grief and bereavement. In: *American Handbook of Psychiatry, Vol. 1,* 2nd ed., ed. S. Arieti. New York: Basic Books, pp. 673–702.

Walker, G. (1991), *In the Midst of Winter*. New York: Norton.

Washington, R. A. (1995), The challenge for behavior science assisting AIDS service organizations to do HIV prevention work. *Psychology & AIDS Exchange,* Fall, pp. 3–4.

Yamamoto, J., Okonogi, K., Iwasaki, T. & Yoshimura, S. (1969), Mourning in Japan. *Amer. J. Psychiat.,* 125:1661.

2 Modifying Psychotherapeutic Methods When Treating the HIV-Positive Patient

Bertram H. Schaffner

In 1984, when I first mentioned to a friend that I was treating an AIDS patient, I was met with the discouraging question, "What is the use of treating such a patient? You can't cure him anyway!" This kind of comment was typical of people who live in a culture imbued with simple standards of success or failure. Also, at that time patients were not identified as having AIDS until extremely far along in the course of the illness and usually did not live long afterward. Fortunately for present-day HIV and AIDS patients, medical treatment has made such strides that they are now living much longer. Consequently, patients need to consider how to improve the quality of their longer life spans, and therapists now have the time to learn more about the special issues that arise for people living with HIV and AIDS and to decide how to meet them.

Theoretically, HIV patients now have sufficient time ahead to work with a therapist. Unfortunately, this is not always the case in real life. In today's world, financial policies and medical administration threaten to limit severely the role of psychotherapy. The HIV patient is often the most affected by such developments. The therapist's task of defining and dealing rapidly with the special psychological needs of HIV patients is daunting. Traditional psychotherapeutic treatment requires many hours, which HIV patients can rarely afford. Therefore, a therapist planning to treat an HIV patient is often obliged to work within a more compressed time frame than he is used to. This is not necessarily easy for him to do. He must modify his treatment to be more topic-focused, on the order of "crisis intervention." To some, the changes outlined in this paper will seem radical.

Many psychotherapists in private practice, and many psychologists, nurses, and social workers who handle a large proportion of the care of HIV patients in hospitals and clinics, have already been quietly modifying their therapeutic approaches. More and more reports of these modifications are being published.

Here are the major differences for the therapist treating the HIV patient:

1. The therapist has to focus on the myriad *external* realities of the patient's life as well as on the *internal.*
2. The therapist is forced to work with special emotional stresses and discomforts that go with the grave unknowns and uncertainties of an HIV patient's life.
3. The therapist is forced to learn about the profound damage inflicted on the HIV patient's life by stigma and how to relieve it. The therapist, as well, often has to learn to live with the stigma that *he too* acquires because he is treating an HIV patient.
4. More than by other illnesses, the therapist is personally challenged and required to reexamine his own values and conceptions about life.

These changes involve shifts in awareness and increased emphasis on uncovering what is uniquely important and meaningful to HIV patients. They also concern the therapist's willingness to deal with awkward, frequently avoided areas, such as gender, death and dying, religion, substance abuse, unconventional sexuality, and other lifestyles.

There is another major change. The therapist treating the HIV patient has to steel himself to the fact that he will be sorely tested with regard to self-revelation. He will be, almost without exception, asked to reveal his own sexual orientation. In traditional Freudian therapy, the therapist strives to remain anonymous and "unknown" to the patient, in order to keep transference issues clear, even though many therapists have doubted whether such a state is actually possible. There is debate at this present time, however, about the potential benefit to the patient from different degrees of therapist self-disclosure. When a therapist elects to use self-revelation, this imposes on him an enormous obligation of self-study in order to know his own values and biases. He must also be sure of his ability to cope with the consequences of self-revelation.

The HIV situation also requires the therapist to play new and unaccustomed roles, such as consultant, teacher, liaison with other medical specialists, family counselor, couples therapist, even policeman. We will examine some of these areas of modification as we go along.

The Initial Interview: The Patient Begins Life Again

In my experience, the initial interview is critically important. In traditional practice, during the first session, a therapist busies himself with obtaining the patient's history, defining the patient's specific areas of neurosis, and making a diagnosis, all the while being sensitive to the patient's reactions to the entire therapeutic situation.

In the initial interview with the HIV patient, the therapist has to place greater emphasis on the current crisis in the patient's life—his present needs and his present vulnerabilities—than on researching his past life and traumas. The therapist must listen carefully to learn the patient's current strengths, assets, and resources.

The first session with an HIV patient is often unforgettable. In my experience, HIV patients frequently have a powerful need to talk, almost without interruption, during the whole first hour. I have wondered what accounts for this special need to talk in this way—a way that requires the therapist to listen especially carefully.

In my mind, it is not the simple result of anxiety. This phenomenon may be due to a number of factors. I feel that the HIV patient is still experiencing the shock of learning his diagnosis, and the realization that his life has been forever changed. I take it for granted that HIV patients are "brokenhearted," and that having come face-to-face with the tragedy of their illness was the most painful moment of their entire lives. Talking at such length may bring the relief that comes from sharing feelings. As an old German proverb states: "Sharing joy doubles joy; sharing grief cuts grief in half."

I believe that in the initial interview, the HIV patient feels impelled to review his entire past life before he became HIV-infected, to survey the present wreckage caused by HIV, and to understand the future difficulties he will face before he can *commit* himself to go on living. Only then can he be ready to contemplate how to live constructively in whatever time will be left.

The Therapist's Special Listening

The grieving HIV patient seeks a therapist for catharsis and validation. He needs the therapist to be a serious and attentive listener who can understand his plight and support him in his future hopes and plans. Nevertheless, despite his need to talk, he may actually have great difficulty in speaking openly about certain aspects of his life because of the danger inherent in revealing unusual lifestyles, sexual activities, and the HIV infection itself. HIV patients often have lived lives of secretiveness and isolation.

At this particularly sensitive juncture, the therapist must insure a therapeutic atmosphere favorable to the patient's talking openly: one that is sympathetic, nonjudgmental, and accepting. Although it is axiomatic that therapists desire always to be sympathetic and nonjudgmental, this may not be the case in matters concerning the HIV patient.

Many HIV patients feel ashamed, undesirable, even unworthy of attention and help. I go out of my way to see that they are treated respectfully by my staff. I have tried to make my office warm and welcoming; this may be easier in my own case, since my office is in my home. I keep complex administrative procedures and frustrating delays to a minimum.

I ease the patient's entry into the therapeutic dialogue by simply asking him to tell me what he wants my help with, in whatever way feels natural to him. I feel there is an important benefit for the HIV patient to know that he retains an active influence on the content of the session.

It is my custom to take verbatim notes of the first interview, because I find that HIV patients tend to reveal the most important clues to their lives in that first session. I find myself reviewing the notes from the first session quite often.

My transcription of sessions seems to help patients in an additional way: many have told me they feel that what they are saying must be important, because I take so much trouble to record it. A few patients have objected to my writing, under the impression that they are not getting my full attention. I assure them that writing actually helps me to concentrate more fully upon them. Especially with HIV patients, I feel that full attention and recording play an important part in restoring their sense of worth as human beings.

A Therapist's Dilemma: To Touch or Not to Touch

Many among my early HIV patients expressed a strong need to be touched, hugged, or held. It seemed to me extremely unlikely that these patients were making sexual overtures. To me it was clear that the combination of fear, physical avoidance, and moral rejection they had experienced since being diagnosed had left them feeling that they were untouchable social pariahs. To me, their desire for physical contact seemed natural, understandable, basically harmless, and theoretically very helpful emotionally. I saw the desire to be touched as need for proof that they were not repulsive to others, or possibly as the need to be comforted, as by a protecting parent. I examined my conduct and I did not find that I had been rejecting or thereby provoking their need for assurance from me. I felt no sexual inclination toward them and was sure of my own ability to respect boundaries. Nevertheless, I was aware that something in me desired to respond to their wishes.

The first encounter with an HIV patient is a highly charged emotional experience. The humanity in all of us is easily drawn to respond compassionately to the tragedy of a patient's situation. Other therapists treating HIV patients have reported similar warmhearted impulses to respond and have expressed concern over what to do about these impulses. We are sometimes tempted to disregard what our previous training and experience have taught us. We may feel at the moment that there is little risk in carrying out a seemingly harmless request for a kind of support that is outside the realm of our normal professional training.

What I am describing took place more often nearly 10 years ago, and prior to more recent widespread public agitation over sexual harassment. At that time what was uppermost was concern about whether touching or hugging a patient would be beneficial or harmful. The chief concerns were potential harm to the transference, and that touching of any kind would be likely to lead to sexual contact. The issue as to whether health-care practitioners can or should try to replace the warm care that is missing in a patient's life has long been controversial; psychotherapists tend to agree that it is unwise and dangerous to attempt this.

I did not change my psychotherapeutic thinking or practice with these patients, yet this issue led me to examine why I had momentarily been inclined to meet a disarmingly simple request. I was relieved when I was able to identify my urge as originating in my early childhood relationship with my mother. She had constantly rewarded me for comforting her in her grief over her own mother's death and in her anxiety over her brother's exposure to mortal danger as a soldier in World War I. I had been tempted, therefore, to respond to my patients as I had been praised for responding to my mother.

Early in the epidemic, such requests from patients to be hugged or touched were fairly frequent. As panic over the illness has decreased and a degree of hopefulness has returned, there has been a parallel reduction in such requests. The few times in 1985 in which I gave encouraging pats on the back or even a reassuring handshake did not seem to harm treatment. It seems preferable, however, to engage the patient in a warm discussion and airing of his feelings and needs and to help him find comfort and reassurance in his ordinary social contacts.

Restoring the Patient's Autonomy and Self-Direction

In working with HIV, the therapist has to keep in mind the importance of restoring a patient's sense of autonomy and self-direction. HIV patients have often lost confidence in their ability to steer their own lives and may feel quite dependent on others. They need to recover faith in their capacity to make decisions and to assume responsibility for themselves. To help them in this, the therapist has to guard against the tendency to overprotect. The harsh realities of HIV patients' lives can understandably tempt a therapist to offer various kinds of assistance, rather than to improve the patients' confidence in their ability to help themselves. As early as the initial interview, I try to bolster patients' confidence in their own judgment.

HIV patients frequently ask the therapist to function as a teacher. They remind me of Chinese and Indian students who often ask at the end of a conversation, "What life lesson should I learn from this?" The therapist, however, must balance the relative value to the patient of preserving his autonomy and self-reliance vis-à-vis the benefits of receiving specific advice. At times, it is indicated and appropriate to function as a teacher. At other times it may be preferable to let the patient know the location and sources of information, so that he can seek it out for himself and arrive at his own conclusions, rather than to provide him with possible answers.

Patients constantly seek the therapist's opinion, not only about psychological matters, but with reference to new medications, diets, holistic medicine, acupuncture, and so forth. There are special dangers for the therapist if he takes on the role of advisor in these areas, which are uncertain, unclear, and where the results of research are inconclusive. The wise therapist will not allow his own preconceptions or preferences to influence the patient's decisions in these areas, despite pressure from the patient. It is better for the patient to take these matters up with his physician.

Rabkin, Remien, and Wilson (1994) have written:

> Expert AIDS physicians hold diverse views and philosophies on treatment. . . . In light of the limited options available in HIV management, the patient may play a greater role in the decision-making process than in other illnesses . . . . Patients, who also differ in their beliefs about treatment strategies, can usually find experienced physicians whose views match their own[p.56].

The patient will often have to draw his own conclusions and make his own decisions.

One does well to remember the incredibly high level of anxiety, concern, and uncertainty with which the HIV patient has to lead his life, and that the psychotherapeutic discussion is the appropriate place to bring these woes. I feel satisfied with the patient's progress when he has come to understand that the ability to tolerate uncertainty is an essential part of emotional maturity. There is also a high demand on the therapist treating an HIV patient to be able to tolerate uncertainty himself.

It is hoped that during this exercise in autonomy and self-direction, both patient and therapist will learn much about living with uncertainty, the ever-present hallmark of the HIV condition.

Relieving Shame: A Special Challenge

Shame is a universal issue among HIV patients, and the therapist is forced to pay special attention to it. Therapists, as well as patients, live in a culture still amazingly prudish and condemning despite progress in "sexual liberation," a culture that stigmatizes diseases connected to sexual activity or substance abuse. HIV patients bear a heavy burden of this shame and disgrace. Shame exists not only in the patient's poor view of himself, but also arises out of the certainty that others also have a low opinion of him. Many patients already live with shame because of their own internalized homophobia or because of inner taboos they have violated; they are now also burdened with additional shame over HIV. As I have already mentioned, the therapists who treat HIV patients discover that a stigma is attached to them as well, simply for providing treatment.

Reduction of shame must be tackled as early as possible, so that the patient can begin to reveal his other problems to the therapist. Untreated shame has serious consequences: despair, depression, self-isolation, withdrawal from therapy, or suicide. No therapist can ignore this task, and it is difficult.

A crucial reducer of shame is the experience of being accepted by a respected authority figure. The therapist hopefully represents such a figure. A sincerely nonjudgmental attitude is a potent factor, especially during the emotional first interview, in lessening the sense of shame over being HIV-positive.

I make special efforts to discuss the patient's life in a calm, constructive, practical way. Many HIV patients have more than one stigma to get over. Therefore I also work with the patient to understand other sources of shame that originated in childhood.

A therapist may accomplish much to improve the patient's self-image in individual therapy. Individual therapy alone, however, may not be sufficient. Especially in the area of shame about HIV, it is often preferable to refer the patient to group therapy, which has proven quite effective in counteracting stigma. Groups provide tangible proof that the patient is not alone and allow him to talk safely with others about HIV and about matters of which he has been too ashamed even to verbalize. Group methods are especially useful when HIV patients begin to resume social life and dating.

The Art of Probing

I now address a specific challenge for the therapist: probing. The therapeutic method requires constant questioning, probing, and challenging of the patient. In the case of HIV patients, this must be done carefully because of their unusual sensitivity to questioning. The patient needs to be sure that the therapist genuinely wants to help him, not just to dissect or expose him. The way the therapist presents his questions is extremely important.

Patients reveal themselves gradually, and only after they have developed sufficient ego strength and trust in the relationship with the therapist. Only then can the therapist begin to ask the patient to explain discrepancies between his thoughts and actions or to explore significant omissions in the descriptions of his life.

Due to the stigma placed on them, as well as to traumatic events in their lives, HIV patients are more likely than others to experience the therapist's questions as critical, accusing, demeaning or dangerous. Such interpretations are more frequent when the patient feels guilty about particular behavior or events that led to his becoming HIV infected.

When questioning an HIV patient, the therapist needs to keep many considerations in mind. On several scores, HIV patients have had to live secret lives. They have suppressed revealing behavior. They have adopted such defense mechanisms as denial and even dissociation in order to keep on functioning. HIV patients, therefore, can be extraordinarily defensive when the therapist's questions provoke fear of the loss of essential confidentiality, as for example, the exposure of a married man's or woman's clandestine extramarital activities and subsequent HIV infection. There is also fear of damaging consequences to a business, military, or political career, or to a living situation should the person's medical status become known.

In the course of treatment I may feel the need to ask questions concerning such sensitive areas, but I am also aware of the patient's resistance to them. At these times, I am faced with the decision of whether to continue my line of questioning, to call attention to the patient's resistance, or to wait. At issue may be the essential question: Is the patient ready to trust me with his secrets or not? The very fact that I bring up an issue will be felt by some patients as pressure.

It is most important at this time for the patient to feel that I am his ally. It is often necessary to win his consent to explore certain areas. If the patient wishes to know the reason for a question, I try to give him a full answer. He then becomes an informed collaborator, but still retains the right to refuse or postpone discussion. I let him know that I am content to postpone an issue, but that I think there is value in dealing with it. Eventually, the patient is likely to return to it of his own accord. The HIV patient needs to feel he is securely in control over perceived dangers.

HIV patients are often confronted with the need to make major changes in their sexual habits. Therapists may find it difficult to ask HIV patients detailed questions about their sexual practices. Investigating these areas is vitally important to the health of the patient and those close to him, as in the issue of "safer sex." It is important not to provoke the patient into resisting or rebuffing the therapist at this point.

In order to enable the HIV patient to talk more candidly about sexual matters, I have found several methods to be useful. I try to use the patient's own vocabulary, rather than impersonal scientific terminology. I try to discuss the issues in a neutral manner, avoiding implications of pathology. I am helped to do this by my assumption that underlying all sexual behavior, including the most bizarre, there is a powerful need for warmth and intimacy. By helping the patient to identify the positive motives that led to his sexual behavior, he will feel freer to discuss it. He will also be more likely to consider alternative, healthier practices to meet his important needs.

I encourage the patient to enter with me upon a joint voyage of discovery, to locate and identify these underlying vital needs. When the needs have been correctly identified, then we can go about reviewing their origins, hopefully helping the patient to understand the true nature of his needs and to revise the unsatisfactory mechanisms by which he had been attempting to fill them.

This essential exploration puts additional pressure on the therapist, who has so much to explore and often little time to do it. I remember, however, Harry Stack Sullivan's concept of a person's inherent "will to health," and it helps me to be patient. It is a slow process to win a defensive patient's consent to be questioned. One must have faith in his eventual willingness to open the door to his inner life.

Unaccustomed Roles for the Therapist

Ordinarily, a psychotherapist functions in a restricted one-to-one relationship with his patient, which makes possible the absolute confidentiality traditionally guaranteed; all other persons are excluded and all transactions take place only between therapist and patient. The realities of HIV illness quickly change this state of total privacy. Frequently, the HIV patient is referred to the therapist by his physician, who already knows about the HIV infection. The internist often needs feedback and recommendations from the therapist to guide him in his management of the patient, especially when there are tensions between patient and internist. If the patient is not helped to resolve friction with his internist, it can affect his compliance with his medical regimen or even induce him to change doctors. In this situation, the therapist is thrust willy-nilly into the role of liaison-consultant. The therapist must also be on the watch for transferential behavior, as for example, when a patient may pit the internist against the therapist or vice versa, much as he may have pitted one parent against the other.

Now the therapist is no longer in a solo relationship with the patient; he has become a part of a "treatment team." This is commonly the case when working with HIV patients. Soon, other members of the treatment team make their appearance. Patients frequently join groups—support, bereavement, caregiver groups—and the therapist will be invited to coordinate his work with that of the group.

Frequently, the relationship between the patient and his partner may be a troubled one. If the patient wants the therapist to meet or work with the partner, the therapist must decide whether meeting the partner (which would have been frowned upon in traditional psychotherapy) will be beneficial, and whether the couple is to undergo couple therapy, either with him or with someone else. I always welcome the opportunity to get to know the partner.

In some cases, the patient requests a change from individual therapy to couple therapy. In the case where they wish to carry out couple therapy with me, I feel it requires extremely careful examination of potential advantages or disadvantages to the ongoing therapy, particularly with regard to the issue of confidentiality. Ordinarily, I prefer to refer them to a couples specialist. In that case, still another person has been added to the treatment team.

The list goes on: members of the patient's biological, legal, and adopted families often become actively involved in the patient's emotional life, financial support, and physical care. From the very beginning, the patient may have profound reservations about whether to inform or involve them at all. The beleaguered HIV patient will usually ask for the therapist's direct help and advice in making such choices. Here, again, the therapist may feel that he could be helpful, but I feel a wise therapist will limit himself to asking the most telling questions to elicit the patient's own store of knowledge about the persons concerned. This will assist the patient to rely upon his own intuitive and critical judgment.

Similar questions will emerge repeatedly, for instance, those regarding the patient's employer, colleagues at work, and social acquaintances. A distressing amount of time may have to be spent responding to comments and criticisms by the patient's family and friends about the therapist himself. This is in addition to the time often demanded by insurance companies, hospital personnel, and other bureaucracies.

Having to function as a member of a treatment team brings not only a change in methodology, it can also cause the psychotherapist some personal distress. First of all, it may be rough on his ego because it diminishes his sense of personal control over the therapeutic situation and exposes his work to the scrutiny and judgment of others, both professionals and laymen. In addition, working with HIV patients forces the therapist to absorb large quantities of new and rapidly changing information, such as advances in treatment, specialized referral lists, safer sex and disease containment methods, familiarity with patients' conflicts concerning HIV testing, HIV-related legal and financial issues, cultural characteristics of various minority groups, community resources. The research required to obtain all this essential background knowledge adds a great deal to the therapist's workload.

In general, HIV illness clearly obliges one to wear many hats and to accept one's poignant limitations in helping other human beings.

Should the Therapist Act as Moral Policeman?

Customarily, the therapist's role is one of maintaining complete neutrality and confidentiality. However, few medical conditions cause a therapist more conflict in this area than those involving prevention of the spread of HIV and the protection of the infected person's sexual partner. When the HIV-negative patient is clearly suicidal or homicidal, the therapist is in difficult but charted territory, with ethical and legal mandates telling him what to do. When an HIV-positive patient puts another person in danger because of unsafe sexual practices, we do not have similarly clear directives.

In such cases, many therapists feel a strong urge to take some kind of action. Most therapists would feel remiss if they did not remind the patient of the moral implications of his actions, and of his ethical obligations to other human beings. Such action might consist of a directive or confrontational approach, with the attendant risk of disrupting the working relationship or the patient even stopping therapy.

Some therapists have consciously avoided exploring the sexual behavior of HIV patients because it is difficult to decide on a course of action once one knows what a patient is doing sexually. And once one knows, it is impossible to "unknow." The therapist's own feelings about the patient's sexual practices have been known to adversely affect the treatment. There is also severe stress for the conscientious therapist because of the conflicting policies of different professional agencies dealing with AIDS, that involve warning a patient's sexual partner.

Historically, people seem to have wanted psychotherapists to function as policemen, as if they actually possessed the power to stop the harmful or self-destructive behavior of their patients. From the beginning of the HIV epidemic, I have been struck by the number of times that professionals, especially early in their work with HIV patients, raise questions about controlling patients who might infect others.

I recognize their concern as extremely important. I understand that in this time of fear it is natural to be preoccupied with preventing the spread of the disease. I myself strongly emphasize teaching "safer sex" measures, making sure that my patients feel responsible for protecting the health of their partners as well as protecting themselves from new and different infections.

I am also puzzled by the fact that a sizable number of my colleagues appear to believe that many HIV patients deliberately set out, almost vengefully, to infect others. Such cases are indeed known; I seriously doubt that they are as frequent as some people fear. I suspect that elements of antihomosexual bias in the general culture may contribute to this suspicion. There is also the possibility that such sexually harmful behavior is projected onto HIV patients, especially males, by persons of either sex who have been physically or emotionally abused.

The essential powerlessness of a therapist to impose immediate changes on patients is a familiar reality. It may nevertheless be hard to accept. The therapist is forced to make delicate decisions, based upon his careful study of the patient's basic personality, on whether and how to apply pressure, however subtle, on the patient. We need to know whether or not a particular patient will rebel, resulting in increased "acting out," or whether he will experience pressure as hostile criticism or as supportive of his strengths. It is important to ascertain when a patient has been behaving carelessly due to a mood disorder, whether his behavior is impulsive or compulsive, or if it was influenced by alcohol or other substances. One must also learn not to expect changes in sexual patterns to come about rapidly, and one must be prepared for relapses. Some therapists have found it effective to use exercises in role-reversal and altruism. It is quite striking to me how often patients have modified careless sexual behavior after I have directly commented on its being selfish or hostile.

In my practice, I try to give my patients the greatest affirmation and credit. I express my admiration for their fortitude and resourcefulness in coping with HIV. Ventilation of their unhappiness, together with my sympathy and recognition for them, I have observed to be quite helpful in bringing about behavioral change, probably much more than I could have accomplished by trying to be a "therapeutic policeman."

Dealing with Dementia

This chapter would not be complete if I failed to mention that frequently during the course of AIDS a patient gradually shows signs of dementia. The patient may become forgetful, confused, and sometimes delusional. He may reach the stage where he cannot correctly identify the people around him. At times he can communicate rationally; at other times he cannot. To the extent that the patient is aware of this deterioration, it can be very frightening.

The therapist must now serve the patient in a new way, as his usual method of verbal and intellectual interchange becomes restricted. The essential emotional aspects of the interpersonal communication with the patient become paramount. The intellectually impaired patient is still able to derive a sense of security from the familiar trusted voice of the therapist. Thus the patient can often be stabilized and reassured by the feeling that his limitations are understood and that he will be taken care of.

In the course of treating HIV patients, both therapist and patient frequently develop a strong personal bond. If the therapist were to interrupt treatment because of the dementia, the patient would feel abandoned. The therapist usually wishes to continue treating the patient through to the end, and may feel guilty of abandonment if he does not. If he continues to the end, the therapist will find himself performing in ways to which he is not accustomed, as a combination of therapist, nurse, interpreter, and friend. Often, at this later stage, the demented patient is no longer able to come to the therapist's office. The therapist may be asked to continue treatment in the patient's home, and must make the often difficult decision of whether or not to do so.

Death and Dying: "Therapist, Know Thyself"

I know of no other illness that so challenges a therapist to know his own deepest beliefs and feelings concerning death and dying as HIV and AIDS. This is the leitmotif that runs beneath nearly everything that transpires between therapist and patient. The essence of helping an HIV patient is to enable him to comprehend the prospect of his own death and to come to terms with it, so that he can live out the rest of his life reasonably at peace, with a sense of some hope and satisfaction. It is of enormous value in helping another human being to cope with the fears and mysteries surrounding death if one has identified one's own feelings about dying and has come to terms with them. However, one's own self-understanding will not be sufficient to give tranquillity to someone else; one needs to familiarize oneself with the many diverse concepts and fears attached to death by different individuals and in different cultures.

Contemporary American secular culture does not automatically provide a clearly formulated spiritual framework for accepting death. American culture places great value on individual life, especially while it is young and healthy. It does not place much value upon human life when it is old or infirm. Most American children are not taught to confront matters connected with death realistically.

Americans have become used to seeing death in the form of exciting entertainment, in itself a denial of the serious reality of it. In addition, many Americans harbor the naive misconception that so-called modern science has basically eliminated the threat of death from everyday life. It is not surprising, therefore, that Americans who are infected with HIV tend to be totally unprepared to deal with the prospect of dying, especially when they are young. HIV patients come into treatment with powerful apprehensions, misconceptions, and expectations that are hard to predict. The therapist comes into the treatment situation with his own set of conscious and unconscious preconceptions. Consequently, the therapist and the patient may both be uncomfortable with the subject of death, though in different ways; this, of course, can interfere with treatment.

Perhaps I can best illustrate this with my experience of not being aware of my own complex feelings, how they took me by surprise, and how my later awareness of them modified my work. I used to feel that I was unperturbed about dying. Originally, when people asked me how I got the courage to treat AIDS patients, I would says "This is what doctors are trained to do," likening the situation to Father Damien and the lepers. Or I would say that I had been lucky in having been taught in early childhood that death is simply a very peaceful "going to sleep," with no frightening references to fire and brimstone in an afterlife.

In August 1944, during World War II, while traveling East across a submarine-infested Atlantic in a troop ship that had lost its convoy and was unprotected from German torpedoes, I was fully aware of a dread of drowning, but I had few fears of dying as such. I calmed whatever fears I had with the thought, "I don't mind dying, as I have really lived; I have loved and have been loved." In the past I had vividly experienced shock and grief over the death of others, such as my grandfather and a close adolescent friend, but I was quite unaware of strong emotions concerning my own possible death. In general, I thought I knew my feelings concerning death, and that I was quite comfortable with them.

However, I was totally surprised 40 years later. In 1984, while I was calmly reading my first paper on AIDS before the American Academy of Psychoanalysis, at the end of the first page I unexpectedly found myself overwhelmed and sobbing, unable to continue. At the time, I did not know why I was weeping, but I knew that it was important for me to find out, and to that end I would have to make a private journey of discovery. There is no single, universal reaction to death; each person's experiences in life determine his unique attitudes toward dying and the death of others. In the course of the last 10 years, and even while preparing this essay, I have uncovered many facets of the puzzle.

My first insight into this incident was that it occurred when I began to speak of the fatigue, sadness, and sense of helplessness among gay doctors who were attempting to save the lives of AIDS patients in that tense early period of the epidemic. I know now that I identified emotionally with both the doctors and the patients, but I had repressed my most intense feelings without knowing why. At that time, I knew only that I profoundly disliked, and tried to avoid expressing, any emotions surrounding death. I was comfortable only with a quiet, so-called philosophical attitude toward death, both my own and others'. Fortunately, I learned that I should struggle to prevent this attitude from creeping into my treatment of patients. I knew that I had to appreciate and respect their grief, and that I should not permit myself, even unconsciously, to attempt to suppress their full outpouring of emotions.

I gradually came to understand that I not only feared but actively resented the emotions surrounding death. I remembered that my mother's mother had died a year before I was born; my mother arrived here shortly afterward, an immigrant in a new country, without an established network of family and friends. Her grief over her mother's death was intense and prolonged. My father, a very reserved man, was not emotionally equipped to help her deal with her feelings. Consequently, my mother poured out her inconsolable grief and rage at God to me and looked to me for emotional support.

But her profound melancholy was too heavy a burden for a child. It left me feeling inadequate to cope with strong expressions of grief, and it left me resentful at being expected to be a parent to my parent. Later I became intolerant of any open demonstration of grief or anger, not only in others but also in myself. Once I became aware of this I could understand my experiencing internally the sadness and pain surrounding death, and my inability to permit myself to express it externally.

The day I read the scientific paper, my feelings of sadness and grief were so strong that they broke through my usual defenses, and I felt ashamed of the loss of control. However, I was surprised and relieved by the audience's warm, positive response and insistence that I complete the reading.

Since that time, tears come to my eyes from time to time while working with HIV patients. Once I would have done my best to hide them, but now I do not find it necessary to do so. Some patients find it to be a welcome and affirming response; none seem to have lost respect for me or to have found it burdensome.

At the age of 84, I now think about my own death frequently and easily. Death will come in its own way and in its own time. I am grateful to have had sufficient time to pursue many of my life goals. I am experiencing the gradual decline in energy and powers that make death the inevitable result of a natural progression.

The HIV patient is clearly less fortunate. He is faced with the task of finding value in a life that will be abbreviated by illness. The therapist must fully grasp the anguish of the HIV patient, who feels profoundly cheated by the curtailment of his life. To combat the patient's bitterness and sense of hopelessness, the therapist needs to remind the patient—who is typically very depressed—of the elements in his life that can still give satisfaction. He needs to counteract the self-disparaging tendencies in the HIV patient, to encourage him to continue to develop and enjoy his potentials now, and to place less emphasis upon what may happen in the future. A therapist's own positive attitude toward life's limitations can be a potent weapon against the patient's sense of futility.

Conclusion

It is obvious that the therapist's task in treating an HIV patient is unusually complex. Many more factors come into play than in other treatments; many more players crowd the stage; the issues that arise are profound and involve every conceivable important aspect of life. The work is extremely demanding. The therapist's own personal maturity is, more than ever, a significant factor in the therapeutic outcome. Because of today's rapidly changing conditions in medical care, it is more necessary than ever to be able to apply psychotherapeutic understanding with little time available to do so.

The therapeutic community has responded to the urgency of the epidemic sympathetically, creatively, unselfishly, and bravely in the face of stigma. For some it has been painful and exhausting. For many of us it has been extraordinarily rewarding. For me it has been a 15-year period marked by tremendous personal growth and the sharpening of my professional skills. My understanding of people and my respect for their flexibility, strength, and courage has deepened enormously. I feel grateful that I had the opportunity to serve other suffering human beings, to repay the debt I owe to the therapists who gave of themselves to help me when I needed them. The epidemic, even with all of its horrors, has provided the motivation and stimulation to our profession to open many doors, and to improve and humanize our ways of helping others.

Reference

Rabkin, J., Remien, R. & Wilson, C. (1994), *Good Doctors, Good Patients.* New York: NCM Publishers.

3 Treatment of Children and Parents in Families with AIDS

Seth Aronson

My life closed twice before its close
It yet remains to see
If Immortality unveil
A third event to me

So huge, so hopeless to conceive
As these that twice befell.
Parting is all we know of heaven,
And all we need of hell.

—*Emily Dickinson*

Some of the ideas concerning the issues of treating parents with HIV/AIDS that are included here arose from a panel I chaired at the Spring 1996 meeting of the American Orthopsychiatric Association in Boston, Massachusetts. I am grateful to Anne Emmerich, M.D., Sandra McLaughlin, L.C.S.W., and José Pares-Avila, M.A., for their participation and comments. Any errors or infelicities are my own.

A loss that is "so huge, so hopeless to conceive" is one that confronts children of parents with AIDS. These children are in the difficult situation of walking a tightrope—on the one hand, continuing the routine of daily life, while on the other, harboring an awareness that within several months or years their parents could die. The shame and stigma that still surround AIDS, as well as other factors to be discussed below, further impinge on the bereavement process of these children.

The confluence of these factors has produced a clinical entity that nearly every mental health professional who deals with youth today will encounter, particularly those working in the public sector. Sadly, it has forced us to reexamine the issue of childhood bereavement through the contemporary lens of HIV and AIDS.

Scope of the Problem

AIDS has become a leading cause of death among Americans aged 25 to 44 (CDC, 1995) and its incidence is markedly rising among women. Many of these women are parents. This has led experts to predict that by the year 2000 there will be approximately 100,000 children orphaned by AIDS in the United States (Levine, 1993); 40,000 of these children will be in New York City. Many other urban centers will be particularly hard hit. Many foster-care and child-welfare agencies have begun organizing specialized boarding units for children who are themselves HIV-infected or whose parents have contracted AIDS. In adults, the comorbidity of HIV and substance abuse has been well documented (CDC, 1995). Children born to substance-abusing parents, therefore, are at risk of contracting HIV. In addition, they may be subjected to developmental-neurological difficulties due to exposure to drugs in utero as a result of their impaired parents' substance use, may suffer abuse and neglect if the parents are incapacitated, and may be exposed to domestic violence (Havens et al., 1995). If we further consider the connection between early object loss and psychopathology, which has been well documented (Bowlby, 1980; Spitz, 1946; Altschul, 1988), we can understand why these children are at great risk and in need of services. Those children who are themselves HIV-infected are also in great need of help, but it is beyond the scope of this chapter to discuss them here. The focus of this chapter is on the clinical issues involved in working with the children of AIDS families, as well as issues in the treatment of the affected parents.

Ironically, children of parents with AIDS remain underserved. This seems to be due, in part, to the fact that they are themselves not medically afflicted, but there is also a resistance to label these children as requiring treatment (Aronson, 1995). Those treating adult patients with AIDS seem to be overwhelmed by the sheer numbers of their caseloads, as well as by the intensity of the work itself. Understandably, they have little energy to devote to the children of their dying patients. Further, the notion of a bereaved, troubled child who has just witnessed the death of a parent after a protracted illness may be too much to bear, even for a seasoned clinician. Consequently, these children do not generally receive the services and treatment they often desperately need.

Issues and Themes in Grief Work with Children of Parents with AIDS

Myriad complicated feelings and needs may be experienced by these children. These include expressions of rage (a common grief response) versus containment of affect; the reconciliation of ambivalent feelings toward the dead or dying parent; the need to transfer positive feelings and attach to new caretakers; and the problem of identifying positively with a parent who is frail, ill, and may have been neglectful of, or abusive toward, the child in the past.

Expression of Rage versus Containment of Affect

Wolfenstein (1969) describes in detail the rage present in bereaved children. They often are angry at the parent for abandoning them through death; they may also feel resentful at having been "marked by destiny" (Szalita, 1974) when compared with more fortunate children. Wolfenstein, Lindemann (1944), Furman (1974), and others describe how this anger at the lost object may be split off and diverted toward the remaining figures in the child's world, such as new caretakers, teachers, or siblings.

Children of parents with AIDS struggle intensely with their rage. All too often they have been neglected or, at times, abused by their parents or their parents' partners. Thus, these children have a great deal of pent-up anger as a result of their past experiences and the loss and abandonment they presently face. In addition, the extended families themselves are often struggling with the loss and have little energy or patience to tolerate or contain a child's display of anger. The message communicated to the child is that family members have exhausted their resources and cannot tolerate any strong displays of affect.

Alternatively, the remaining family members may be enraged at the child's parent for contracting AIDS, using drugs, or being homosexual, and will brook no discussion about the loss. Their own rage leads to a stifling of any expression of feeling on the child's part. These children then learn that they must silently, privately mourn their parent and consequently turn their feelings inward. The shame connected with having lost a parent to AIDS is further reinforced by the silence that is imposed on the child by the family.

The child's rage may be further compounded by his or her frustration with a parent's drug use and associated neglect. Althea, a 13-year-old girl, recounted how she would attempt to throw out or hide her mother's needles. Nevertheless, her mother, despite being HIV-infected and ill, would conceal some needles from Althea so that, inevitably, she could satisfy her craving for heroin. Althea described how her frustration with her mother's lack of regard for her health led Althea to rageful crying fits and arguments with her ill mother.

In other instances, a parent may have contracted AIDS through sexual contact. Despite the natural parent's drug-free lifestyle, the choice of a substance-using, at times abusive partner may lead to rageful feelings in the child. Sapphire's searing novel, *Push* (1996), portrays a girl in early adolescence who discovers she is HIV-positive after having been raped for years by her mother's boyfriend. She rails against her mother for allowing such a man into their home and destroying the fabric of their lives.

Such rage is often manifest in behavioral difficulties and fighting in school. A disproportionate anger may be displayed in the classroom, with peers, or at home, echoing Lindemann's (1944) notion of the displacement of the anger resulting from grief.

Ambivalence

Szalita (1974) compares the process of mourning to the analysis of transference. In both instances, the patient struggles to forego a dependence on parental figures and integrate ambivalent feelings.

Bereaved children must ultimately disengage from the dead parent, work through the idealization of the lost object (Wolfenstein, 1966), and arrive at an integrated, coherent representation of the parent. As Loewald (1962) writes, "mourning involves not only the gradual, piecemeal relinquishment of the lost object, but also the internalization, the appropriation of aspects of this object" (p. 493).

But how does a child "appropriate aspects" of a parent who has abandoned her by way of illness and death and who may have provided her with a life of abuse and neglect? The child, grappling with conflicted images of the parent while concurrently being exhorted by relatives to express only sorrow, finds such an appropriation a particularly daunting task.

The reconciliation of the ambivalence may depend, not only on the child's achieved level of object relations, but also on pressure to conform to cultural norms of bereavement. Yesenia, a nine-year-old girl, wept openly in session. Her mother, blind, weak, and demented, was dying of AIDS. Yesenia felt only sorrow and pity for her. However, this same woman would beat Yesenia with a broom handle so severely that several times child welfare agencies removed her from her mother's home. Yesenia's tears were from frustration: "What do I do about all those horrible times when she hit me? I think about them as I look at her lying in bed. I can't tell the nurse, she'll think I'm awful. I don't know what to do," she sobbed.

A further complication in the reconciliation of the ambivalence may result for the child who has been raised in a single-, rather than a two-parent, family. Much of the literature on childhood bereavement presumes the existence of a surviving parent. For children of parents with AIDS, that is often not the case. Faced with the thought of losing the only parent, the child may be unable to tolerate any negative feelings about the parent; this makes the negotiation of a clear, cohesive, and integrated representation of the parent nearly impossible. On the other hand, having two parents may permit the child to fully explore ambivalence, not engage in splitting, and emerge with an integrated picture of the ill parent.

José, 12, was living with his father. His mother, who had AIDS, left him when he was eight because she was unable to care for him owing to her substance abuse. José's father was quite supportive of him. As a result, in sessions José was able, with some difficulty, to explore his highly polarized feelings about his mother. He recalled happier times when he and his mother would go to the beach, but also acknowledged his anger and disappointment at his mother for her drug use and subsequent abandonment of him.

Transfer of Positive Feelings and Attachment to New Caretakers

It is critical for bereaved children to have caring, supportive figures who will provide for them. This new relationship must be secure enough so that the child may ultimately develop constructive identifications with the lost parent, while progressing in development. The support provided may come literally in the form of food and shelter as well as maintenance of a sense of self.

Children of parents with AIDS often experience significant breaches in support. They may be shuttled between family members as their parents are periodically hospitalized. Additional upheavals may occur in the form of abrupt changes in schools, neighborhoods, and living conditions. It is not uncommon for children to be sent off to another city, state, or country to live with relatives they often don't know. These sudden, disorienting changes may force the child to steadfastly maintain a psychological tie to the dead parent at the expense of a more solid attachment to new caretakers. These all-too-frequent hiatuses in attachment may leave the child in a "developmental vacuum" (Nagera, 1970) with tenuous sources of support for food, clothing, and a sense of continuity.

Recent explorations of attachment have demonstrated its importance for development of sense of self, as well as for promoting object relations (Fonagy, 1993). The breaches in attachment these children experience impede the growth of a stable sense of self while doing little to foster trust and faith in the presence of the other. Their style of attachment can be quick, indiscriminate, and fleeting. Selena, an eight-year-old girl, went to greet the male therapist with a hug. Her mother, in an advanced stage of AIDS, informed the therapist of her concern that Selena often wishes to sit in the laps of adults she hardly knows. Selena repeated her requests to sit in the therapist's lap, although it was clear that she did not know the therapist's name.

Problems of Identification

Many writers (Loewald, 1962; Wolfenstein, 1966, 1969; Szalita, 1974; Pollock, 1978) discuss the importance of identifying with the dead parent so as to psychologically incorporate aspects of the lost object and continue with future attachments. For children of parents with AIDS, this identification can be hampered by various factors.

Young children struggling with issues of body integrity may be frightened by their parents' physical deterioration. If their self-other differentiation is not fully developed, fantasies of being infected or afflicted themselves may ensue. Raquel and Shaquanna, two sisters aged 9 and 11, spoke of their abject terror upon visiting their hospitalized mother. She lost her sight and had become incontinent. "She's not the mommy we know," they cried. They began to wonder if they too would become blind, despite the knowledge that neither of them was HIV-infected.

This fear can be exacerbated if the parent becomes demented, resulting in the child's fantasies of "going crazy."

Familial rage at the parent for past drug use, promiscuity, or a homosexual life style may also seriously affect the child's attempts at identification. Similarly, the extended family may actually connect the child with the parent in a negative way, fostering a less than optimal identification. One grandmother brought her six-year-old grandson to the clinic. Her chief complaint was that Malik was playing with dolls. Further questioning revealed that Malik's father, who was bisexual, had died of AIDS. The grandmother's concern was that Malik's doll play was a sign of homosexuality and that he would "turn out like his father." Treatment then focused on her understanding of appropriate developmental norms for play, broadening her sense of gender stereotypes as well as helping her to begin to portray Malik's father in a more positive light.

Treatment Considerations: Child

Two important prerequisites for successful grief resolution have been noted in the literature: one is the availability of a parental substitute with whom the child may forge a new connection; the other is the establishment of a positive, constructive identification with the lost parent (Wolfenstein, 1966, 1969). Toward this end, work with the new caretakers is critical in helping them to understand the child's bereavement process, to create an open environment in which questions can be asked and feelings expressed, and, ultimately, to foster a new attachment.

Nurturing the new attachment involves work with both child and caretaker. Many of these caretakers are grandparents who may require a good deal of support around the issues of raising young children or adolescents later in life. They also may need to be reminded of the importance of portraying their sons and daughters in a positive light to the child, despite the grandparents' anger at their children for many years of conflict.

Phillip's grandmother initially would not tolerate any mention of Phillip's mother's name. Her daughter had a long history of truancy, drug use, and theft, and had served time in prison. Yet it became clear that Phillip needed to have some comforting memories of his mother and, over time, the grandmother was helped to recount positive anecdotes about her daughter, once she realized the importance for her grandson.

Oftentimes, the clinician must work with outside agencies, such as school or foster-care agencies, to ease the child's transition and allow for new attachments.

The burgeoning "permanency-planning" movement represents an effort to help the child move as seamlessly as possible to a new home. Permanency planning allows the dying parent to plan for the child and name the child's guardian. Consequently, the child can begin to spend time with the new guardian, enjoying overnight stays and outings, all in the hope of fostering a new attachment. Work with the parent concerning who the best provider or guardian will be allows the dying parent to feel some sense of mastery, as well as a feeling that the child will be provided for after the parent's death.

The child's ambivalence toward the parent with AIDS should be worked through to some sense of resolution. Such resolution then permits the child to connect with new caretakers. This is no small task. Often it involves recognition and acceptance of anger toward the parent as well as a diminishing of externalization. The anger toward the parent for abandonment through death must be acknowledged and resolved, rather than displaced.

In one group for children of parents with AIDS, early sessions were focused on the children's rage at politicians for not spending enough money on AIDS research. Over time, the youngsters were helped to see that, politics aside, it was not the mayor or president with whom they were angry (or the nurse and doctor who could not save their parents), but their parents themselves for having contracted the virus.

Helping families to create an atmosphere of open communication is critical. Despite our best efforts at education, there remains a stigma and an air of secrecy around AIDS, of which these children are all too aware. The emotional valence of the issue further confounds the child's inability to cognitively assimilate and master information.

A clinician began consulting in an urban junior high school shortly after the entire school had participated in AIDS Awareness Week, complete with educational and informational programming. Many students were still reluctant to ask questions, and those that did were clearly confused about elementary issues regarding AIDS, unprotected sex, and so forth. One girl wondered if a condom would prevent her getting cancer from a sexual partner. Another boy was afraid to let his cousin (who was HIV-positive) touch him for fear of contracting AIDS. It was only after additional educational sessions that these children could begin to process their emotional responses to their home situations.

The adults in these families, then, must permit open discussion, questions, and expression of feelings, which can be further reinforced by the therapist. It is only through the initial cognitive mastery of the facts surrounding a loss and subsequent understanding of the human response to loss that a sense of shame and isolation can be diminished and an acceptance and working through of the tragic event of a parent's death can be achieved.

Treatment Considerations: Parent

Just as the child faces issues regarding attachment, resolution of anger, and establishment of open communication (among others), so, too, does the HIV-infected parent.

The attachment of parents to their children may be affected by numerous factors. Many HIV-infected parents who bring their children for treatment want help in disclosing their illness to their children. Such disclosure is fraught with conflict: What will the child's response be? Will it affect their relationship with the child? Often parents fear that after disclosing to the child, the child will in turn (purposefully or inadvertently) inform relatives, teachers, or neighbors, perhaps bringing the wrath of the various systems (e.g., school, child welfare) down on the family and fracturing the household. Unfortunately, there is an all-too-real basis for such fears. David Kirp (1989) recounts the responses of America's schools to children and families with AIDS. Too often, children of parents with AIDS have been stigmatized and isolated through a perverse notion of "guilt by association." Disclosing the nature of the illness may also stir feelings in the parent that counteract the adaptive use of denial, and may elicit enormous anxiety about death and dying—anxiety that may be debilitating for the parent.

Luisa, a 34-year-old mother of two, presented for treatment with the dilemma of whether or not to disclose her HIV status to her 12-year-old son, Jonathan. She felt that each day she kept this information from him, they grew further apart and she feared the distance growing between them. In individual parent sessions, the exploration (and projection) of her fears were examined. After several weeks, joint parent-child sessions were held in which Luisa was able to disclose her condition to her son.

Such disclosure may also lead to discussion of previous or hidden lifestyle choices. A parent with a long past history of IV drug use may be uncomfortable dredging up painful memories in a candid discussion with his or her children. Such parents also may fear that their histories or lifestyles may lead their children to reject them, which can be especially frightening when faced with the prospect of long and protracted illness and a need for familial support.

Jocalinda's father requested an individual session for himself. He had been caring for her since she was a toddler when her drug-addicted mother fled the city. Recently diagnosed with HIV, he feared telling

Jocalinda about his homosexuality, believing that this would lead her to recoil from him. Parent sessions were focused on his own feelings about his sexuality, which needed to be addressed prior to disclosing his HIV status to his 13-year-old daughter. Eventually, this man was able to speak openly with his daughter about his homosexuality, which she accepted with virtually none of the reservations he had feared.

Further complications affecting attachment include the parent's actual symptoms, such as fatigue or opportunistic infections, that may preclude extensive physical contact with the child. Aside from the actual physical symptoms, the sheer number of medical appointments and the psychic preoccupation these involve may also influence the amount of time and energy the parent has to spend with the child.

Parents' rage at having contracted AIDS will also affect their connection to their children. Many parents, upon initial diagnosis, are so enraged that they have little thought for anyone else. This rage may turn into frustration with their own lives and with choices they have made.

A parent may handle this anger in various ways. Some parents institute a regime of harsh discipline and strict curfews for their children; they are determined that their children not make the same mistakes. Any signs that children are interested in anything that could lead to HIV infection, such as sex or drug use, is met with swift disapproval and discipline. This is particularly true for those HIV-infected parents with adolescent children. The teenager's burgeoning sexuality often evokes fear in a parent that through a careless mistake, the child could become infected as well. Family life can be markedly disrupted by arguments over boy- or girlfriends, sexual activity, or experimentation with any drug. As a result, at a time when attachment should be intensified, parents and adolescents often find themselves very much at odds with each other.

Other parents begin to harbor jealousy of their children's youth, vitality, and opportunity for a healthy, long life. The sight of their vivacious, playful children only reinforces for them their sense of impending mortality. In parent-child sessions, Maria snapped at her young children whenever they took out a new toy. She yelled at them for playing too loudly. When the therapist questioned her, she said, "What do they care—they're young and healthy. But who will take care of me when I'm sick?"

In each case, individual attention must be paid to the parent's needs, so that, in turn, they can effectively parent their own children. Such an understanding echoes Fraiberg's (1975) pioneering work of treating the child through treatment of the parent.

Just as the children of these families require a sense of open communication, so, too, do the parents. Many HIV-infected parents have a plethora of questions: What do I tell the school? The babysitter? The extended family? Treatment can be used to rehearse discussions with the various figures in both the child's and parent's life to alleviate anticipatory anxiety.

Imber-Black, Roberts, and Whiting (1988) have noted the significance of rituals for families. Parents can be helped to create their own kinds of legacies for their children, be they in the form of letters, videos, or mementos put aside for their children. Such actions can be extremely powerful and evocative, often helping parents to come to terms with their illness in ways that simple words could not. Chris, an engaging, impish eight-year-old boy, spoke often of how physically powerful his father had been prior to his illness ("He was diesel, man!"). He proudly showed the therapist photos of his father lifting weights. These photographs, given to him by his father before his death, provided Chris with an important focus for positive memories of his father's strength and vitality at times when Chris was overwhelmed by his father's present debilitated condition.

HIV-infected parents may also fear infecting their children and take unnecessarily strict precautions. This may occur even when the parent is thoroughly educated regarding risk of transmission. In the case of faulty knowledge about HIV transmission, it may be incumbent upon the therapist to educate the parent (and child) about risk factors. Often, however, this fear is related to the parent's own personal sense of shame and stigma, which can be addressed therapeutically. The clinician may note how these unnecessarily strict precautions might represent the parent's feeling that he or she is tainted, dirty, or a contaminant, which might have the unfortunate secondary result of creating distance between parent and child.

For those who contracted the illness through substance abuse, the initial diagnosis is a time of great risk. Many parents express the wish to shoot up again in order to escape the painful reality of an HIV diagnosis. Attendance at Alcoholics Anonymous or Narcotics Anonymous can be a useful adjunct support at this critical point. Infected parents must also combat wishes to withdraw from their children, which may stem from a belief that such withdrawal will ultimately make the final separation less painful. Such wishes can be addressed individually with the parent, so that the parent can be helped to see the defensive nature of such an act as well as its implications for attachment to the child.

There are times when families affected by AIDS present with the children running amok. In such instances, it may not only be parental fatigue that prevents firmer discipline and limit-setting, but also guilt at having to enforce limits that may detract from the small amount of quality time ("precious moments") that is left.

Finally, HIV-infected parents have very real medical considerations that may limit and affect involvement in their children's lives. Fatigue, medical appointments, hospitalizations, all will necessarily impinge on the time and energy a parent may have to offer. School personnel were angry with Serena's mother for her lack of involvement in her daughter's academics. One day, an ambulance pulled up in front of the school and Selena's mother, aided by a nurse and helped to breathe with an oxygen mask, emerged. She had been unable to attend a parent-teacher conference up until then, but wanted to make an appearance to demonstrate her desire for involvement.

Alternative Types of Treatment Modalities

Aside from individual and family therapies, group treatment has been shown to be an effective modality in working with children of parents with AIDS (Aronson, 1994). Support groups for both children and parents can help to alleviate the sense of aloneness that is reported by many who are affected by AIDS. Group work has the further benefits of creating a sense of universality (Yalom, 1975), which is a sense that there is a commonality of feelings and responses to the difficulties involved. Such universality certainly helps to decrease the sense of shame, isolation, and stigma.

As noted above, collateral work with the parents and caretakers is an integral part of the treatment process. The new caretakers, often the grandparents, have their own developmental life-phase issues that need to be addressed, in addition to the difficulties of raising a bereaved child while struggling with their own sense of loss. They may harbor resentment toward their ill son or daughter for the imposition of having to raise a child later in life. It may be necessary to provide support to the caretakers concerning child-rearing issues as well as to explain the various ways in which children express grief.

One grandmother brought her seven-year-old granddaughter in for treatment, complaining, "She doesn't cry or nothing. Her mother died and no tears!" Instead, the girl secreted and hoarded food in her room, which infuriated the grandmother. Over time, the symbolic nature of the child's actions was explained as a manifestation of grief and deprivation, and as a consequence there was a lessening of the grandmother's anger.

New configurations of families have forced clinicians to examine their modes of working and to be creative about who they include in treatment and when. A flexibility and fluidity may be called for, such as seeing a child individually, a parent individually, or having several parent-child sessions. In essence, each family will present with its own set of issues that must be dealt with in a creative and, above all, a respectful manner.

A Look to the Future

It is clear that the number of children whose lives are affected by AIDS is growing (CDC, 1995). There is a need for increased identification of these children (and their families) because they are at risk of psychological difficulties resulting from the many adversities they face. Work with schools, hospital clinics, and foster-care agencies must become more comprehensive and extensive in helping to identify these children in need.

Anna Freud's (1951) pioneering work with child survivors of the Holocaust represented one of the first efforts to develop a model for work with children who were affected by a pressing, contemporary issue. As this decade draws to a close, we must develop our own integrated models for serving youth and families affected by the current problems of the day, in particular HIV and AIDS. "One-stop shopping" models are being developed that provide medical, psychological, social, and even legal services to these families in one location, which fosters a strong connection between the helping professional and the family, while concurrently making it easier for families to receive services. These centers are generally hospital-based, which allows for easy access to medical and dental care (the latter often a problem for patients with AIDS), and are often funded by grants, such as the federally funded Ryan White Title I Act (Keane, 1996; Emmerich, McLaughlin, and Pares-Avila, 1996; Havens et al., 1995). It is critical that these centers, formed around the delivery of mental health services, continue to receive monies, because their access to resources and trained personnel helps to foster a strong connection between the family and the helping professional.

In her famous diary, recounting the years during which she and her family hid from the Nazis, Anne Frank (1952) wrote, "When will we be granted the privilege of smelling fresh air? And because I must not bury my head in the blankets, but the reverse . . . I must keep my head high and be brave, the thoughts will come, not once, but oh, countless times. Believe me, if you have been shut up for a year and a half, it can get too much for you some days" (p. 111). A challenge remains for clinicians who work with children of families with AIDS today. While we acknowledge that "it can get too much . . . some days," we must understand that these children can be helped to keep their heads high and ultimately to grieve in a manner that allows them to continue with the developmental tasks of childhood.

References

Altschul, S., ed. (1988), *Childhood Bereavement and Its Aftermath.* Madison, CT: International Universities Press.

Aronson, S. (1994), Group intervention with children of parents with AIDS. *Group,* 18:133–140.

——— (1995), Five girls in search of a group. *Internat. J. Group Psychother.,* 45:223–235.

Bowlby, J. (1980), *Attachment and Loss, Vol. 3.* New York: Basic Books.

CDC: Centers for Disease Control and Prevention (1995), *HIV/AIDS Surveillance Report,* 7(2).

Emmerich, A., McLaughlin, S. & Pares-Avila, J. (1996), Clinical observations from the treatment of parents infected with HIV: Major psychosocial concerns and implications for treatment. Presented at American Orthopsychiatric Association spring meeting, Boston.

Fonagy, P. (1993), Psychoanalytic and empirical approaches to developmental psychopathology: An object relations perspective. *J. Amer. Psychoanal. Assn.,* 41:245–260.

Fraiberg, S. (1975), Ghosts in the nursery. *J. Amer. Acad. Child Psychiat.,* 14:387–422.

Frank, A. (1952), *The Diary of a Young Girl.* New York: Simon & Schuster.

Freud, A. (1951), An experiment in group upbringing. *The Psychoanalytic Study of the Child,* 6:127–168. New York: International Universities Press.

Furman, E. (1974), *A Child's Parent Dies.* New Haven, CT: Yale University Press.

Havens, J., Mellins, C., Ryan, S. & Locker, A. (1995), Mental health needs of children and families affected by HIV/AIDS. In: *Mental Health Services for HIV-Affected Populations in New York City,* ed. P. G. Goldstein, H. Goodman & G. Landsberg. New York: Coalition of Voluntary Mental Health Agencies, pp. 25–43.

Imber-Black, E., Roberts, J. & Whiting, R., eds. (1988), *Rituals in Families and Family Therapy.* New York: Norton.

Keane, T. (1996), Considerations in the mental health care of children/adolescents affected by HIV/AIDS. Presented at American Orthopsychiatric Association spring meeting, Boston.

Kirp, D. (1989), *Learning by Heart America's Communities.* New Brunswick, NJ: Rutgers University Press.
Levine, C. (1993), *Orphans of the HIV Epidemic.* New York: United Hospital Fund.
Lindemann, E. (1944), Symptomatology and management of acute grief. *Amer. J. Psychiat.*, 101:141–148.
Loewald, H. (1962), Internalization, separation, mourning and the superego. *Psychoanal. Quart.*, 31:483–504.
Nagera, H. (1970), Children's reactions to the death of important objects: A developmental approach. *The Psychoanalytic Study of the Child*, 25:360–400. New York: International Universities Press.
Pollock, G. (1978), Process and affect: Mourning and grief. *Internat. J. Psycho-Anal.*, 59:255–276.
Sapphire (1996), *Push.* New York: Knopf.
Spitz, R. (1946), Anaclitic depression. *The Psychoanalytic Study of the Child*, 2:313–342. New York: International Universities Press.
Szalita, A. (1974), Grief and bereavement. In: *American Handbook of Psychiatry*, Vol. 1, 2nd ed., ed. S. Arieti. New York: Basic Books, pp. 673–684.
Wolfenstein, M. (1966), How is mourning possible? *The Psychoanalytic Study of the Child*, 21:93–123. New York: International Universities Press.
——— (1969), Loss, rage and repetition. *The Psychoanalytic Study of the Child*, 24:432–460. New York: International Universities Press.
Yalom, I. (1975), *The Theory and Practice of Group Psychotherapy.* New York: Basic Books.

4 Gidget Goes to Sing-Sing

An Interpersonal Therapeutic Approach to HIV-Positive Substance Abusers

Susan Bodnar

I was hired to develop and then run an outpatient psychotherapy program at St. Clare's Hospital in New York City. It specialized in the treatment of disenfranchised persons with HIV and AIDS. My first days at work were difficult. Patients crowded the dusty waiting room, leaning listlessly into the blue plastic chairs screwed to the floor. Soap operas blared on a large television suspended from the ceiling. When I asked for my patient schedule, the receptionist bellowed out into the waiting room, "Hey, does anyone out there want to see a psychologist?" Multiple-drug-resistant tuberculosis was rampant. An HIV-negative physician had just died from it.

My patient population included many persons who identified themselves as belonging to racial and cultural minorities. Many had been without resources most of their lives. Others had become impoverished since becoming ill. Only a few were middle class. Some were drug dealers, some were drag queens, and some were priests. Being good at whatever they did was something they shared. No matter what their context, they were its stars.

Almost 45 percent had contact with mental health services through prison or drug-treatment centers, 45 percent had never had exposure to psychotherapy, and the remaining 10 percent had ongoing ties to mental health services. Close to 70 percent had criminal drug records. Over 90 percent came from substance-abusing families. The percentage of exposure to domestic violence as well as to childhood physical and sexual abuse was equally as high. I had to learn a different psychotherapy.

A large percentage of these people struggled with sexual preference and gender identity. At times, it felt as though the hospital were a set for the film *Paris Is Burning.* Initially, I referred to one of my transvestite patients as "he." I was corrected vehemently. "It's she," she chided. The next time I had a transvestite patient, I referred to him as "her" only to be scolded again. This "he" wasn't a "she." He was a "him" just doing "her." Sometimes he was a she and at other times she was a he, and butch queens and femme queens weren't the same as gay men who were butch or femme, and semibutch queens were another category of transvestite altogether. I had to learn a new language.

I encountered difficulties trying to set up a therapeutic frame. For example, before starting sessions with patients presently incarcerated, a security guard first unlocked their wrist and ankle chains. The guard then made himself comfortable in a seat just outside the door that was kept ajar. Regulations required that the prisoner be in sight of the guard at all times. Each and every time, I explained the competing laws governing confidentiality. Some guards complied with my request for a closed door. Some argued. Some thought I was foolish. Simply sitting with my patient was a diplomatic feat. The barriers that had been erected to protect the citizen from the criminal inadvertently distinguished the living from the dying. To speak to one another, my patient and I crossed a divide. Crossing into each other's territory meant momentarily suspending the identities of psychologist and prisoner. I had to learn to cross new frontiers.

Everything seemed to take on the color of the therapeutic mission. My office, located in the hospital attic, had a terrace that doubled as a pigeon burial ground. Even the birds were dying. Drag queen or drug abuser, even an exuberant psychologist in her first job, we shared a common goal. Death was a great humanizer. When someone stopped showing up in the waiting room we knew why. I don't know if Sullivan's (1953) assertion of our common humanity was grounded in the reality of death, but I found myself thinking how true it is that we are all more human than otherwise. I had to learn new—and uncomfortable—truths.

Creating an Alliance

Establishing a therapeutic alliance was complicated by my patients' difficulty with intimacy and by my own countertransference. I found that the patients had at least three obstacles to closeness. The first was HIV disease, or an AIDS diagnosis. Significant others often avoid persons with HIV and AIDS. The patients consequently experience social isolation. They also fear infecting others. The mythical metaphor for intimacy, "the blood brother," becomes a potentially deadly fraternity.

My patients' childhood histories caused a second difficulty with intimacy. Most had experienced trauma in early relationships, disruptions in parental care, and irregular nurturing. Early on they had developed distorted attachments to others. They pursued these attachments into adulthood. They often sought intimacy in a utilitarian fashion. Troubled people of all genders and classes characteristically identified with deviance. Sexual and drug activities were a tolerable form of human contact for persons who believed themselves to be socially marked as abnormal. An HIV diagnosis interrupted the addictive behaviors that were often their only reference for relatedness.

Another problem with intimacy was that many people with whom I worked had achieved the social status of "liminality," a term coined by anthropologist Victor Turner (1969).

> The attributes of liminality or of liminal personae ("Threshold people") are necessarily ambiguous, since this condition and these persons elude or slip through the network of classifications that normally locate states and positions in cultural space. Liminal entities are neither here nor there; they are betwixt and between the positions assigned and arrayed by law, custom, convention, and ceremonial [p. 95].

These people believed themselves to be outsiders, loners, and mavericks. Many had constructed "alternative" communities and had even achieved some context-bound successes within them. Much to their credit, they avoided becoming psychiatric patients. Their neither-here-nor-there status, not quite in but never fully out of our cultural mainstream, was further emphasized by their HIV diagnosis. They didn't quite possess life's possibilities, but they weren't quite dead yet.

To further complicate the liminal experience, people with HIV and AIDS are aware of their role in the AIDS drama of our culture. The AIDS crisis exposes sexual preferences, substance abuse, and death. The current cultural mainstream can no longer deny that human beings have sex with all kinds of other human beings, that they use drugs, and that they die. The exposure of previously taboo behaviors has generated significant group process and ensuing political activity. When an individual's disease becomes an issue for the White House or ACT-UP, the personal experience of people with HIV and AIDS can get lost. I came to agree with psychologist James Hillman (1996) that psychotherapeutic interventions need to facilitate a person's return to the self.

As if *their* problems with intimacy weren't enough, *I* struggled with my own countertransference problems. There are obvious difficulties inherent in spending so much time with death. Like many people in the AIDS field, I was receptive to accepting a job in this field because I had been exposed to loss; my husband of eight years had recently died of cancer. Familiar with the range of emotions and behaviors loss can induce, I could be open and respectful to the experiences of patients and their families, and remain relatively calm during dramatic and difficult crisis points. Yet for me, doing the work meant living with an ongoing sadness and the suspension of hope for a cure. This led to professional angst as well as depression.

I found it difficult to cope with maladaptive behaviors that upset and bothered me. Some of the people with whom I worked committed crimes, they hurt and sometimes killed other people. They neglected their children. They attempted to manipulate me for drugs.

Milagros, a 29-year-old Hispanic woman hospitalized with multiple-drug-resistant tuberculosis, told me that she used to shoot cocaine while pregnant. She said she could feel her unborn child kick and squirm as the cocaine entered her bloodstream. When I heard this, I wanted to scream. I was horrified.

José, a 31-year-old Puerto Rican man, was a member of a motorcycle gang. For many months he was also a twice-a-week psychotherapy patient. During one session he told me the degree of violence to which he had been exposed. He brought a large knife to the next session. I was scared. When another patient, Leroy, asked me in my isolated attic office near the pigeon memorial terrace, "What if I am a rapist?" a deep chill went down my spine.

I learned to use anger, fear, and antipathy. My feelings kept me sane. They functioned as an alarm system and helped me pace myself. When necessary, they led me to dash to the local expensive Italian restaurant for lunch.

My feelings also kept me close to patients who knew how socially maladjusted their behavior had been. To remain impassive when a patient discussed behavior he or she knew to be willfully wrong and abusive would be disrespectful.

My feelings kept me humble. I was not going to cure character disorder or AIDS. My goals became simple: help people get into good relationships, maintain friendships, mend broken family ties, and do some work of which they could be proud. My therapeutic challenge was to design a therapeutic program that would respect the patient's liminal status. At the same time I wanted to challenge it by exciting curiosity. I wanted the people who participated in the program to think about the interaction of their medical diagnosis and their personality function.

The Use of the Self in the Enterprise of Creating an Effective Working Alliance

As I struggled to figure out how people who feared and mistrusted one another could build a therapeutic alliance, I thought about "otherness," the anthropological term for people outside of one's cultural reference points.

I wasn't sure whether they or I were more "other," but I tried to practice the kind of participant observation I had learned in my training, first in anthropology and later in psychology. I got to know my patients. I chatted with them and asked them to draw me pictures of their families. I set up community meetings to find out what services they needed and to include their input in designing the program. Most importantly, I let them get to know me.

I let my emotions show when Milagros told me her story. She was moved by my reaction, and could then share her own self-hatred and her anguish about being responsible for her child's stillbirth. Finding a way to speak together became instrumental in figuring out how to form an alliance.

When José brought his knife to session, I got angry at him for symbolically threatening our relationship. "You know that bringing a knife here would upset me," I told him. "Why would you want to do that?" He was surprised. The attempt to process my feelings with him snuffed out the drama he had kindled.

To Leroy I was more direct: "If you are a rapist, we'll talk about it. It would be hard for me, and I might be frightened, but I can try to listen to you and understand you. But if you are trying to intimidate me, it will surely work, and you will not have a psychologist anymore." He smiled with what seemed like respect. He never tried to frighten me again. He was, in fact, a convicted rapist. We had much to work through, given our differences in status and the racial factors that underlay these differences.

The importance of letting my patients get to know me was underscored when I overheard some inmates and staff joking about "Gidget."[1] It seemed the patients had labeled my arrival at the hospital "Gidget Goes to Sing-Sing." After nine years of analysis and 27 years of education, I was ready to be Dr. Bodnar. I denied that there was a Gidget component to my personality. I felt devalued and defensive.

Yet by giving me this nickname, my patients were taking me in and trying to make sense of my peripheral presence in their lives. What might have been my counterphobia, or my resolute determination to succeed at my first job out of training, was experienced as fresh, innocent, and very much alive. Furthermore, I had always thought of myself as an "other." In their eyes, I was the mainstream. I was what they weren't or couldn't be, what they wanted yet rejected.

I certainly didn't want to be Gidget, but I had to acknowledge the Gidget parts of myself and create the honesty necessary for a therapeutic alliance. Gidget became a symbol in an incipient shared system of meaning (Geertz, 1973). Their fantasies of me—my white clapboard house with the green lawn, the Lamborghini my father had given me for my 16th birthday, and what white girls were like in bed—reminded me of how toys are used in play therapy. We used these fantasies to talk about each other, and as Gidget became real for me, I could become more real for them as someone who could be grabbed onto, hopefully, to facilitate psychological growth.

Creating Chumship

Having found some reasonable basis for a working alliance, I was able to address the loneliness and isolation of some of the people with whom I worked. Aware that Sullivan (1953) considered childhood chumship[2] to be a useful developmental step for the acquisition of personal efficacy, I used groups to create a friendship system. The groups were run by various staff members whom I trained. The staff members designed groups that reflected their interests. A lesbian ran the women's group. A recovering alcoholic ran the recovery group. An older man ran the men's group. A Latino gay male ran a gay-men-of-color group. I filled in with the beginner's group and a spirituality

1. Gidget was a character in a popular American television show from the late 50s and early 60s. She was young, energetic, and morally sanguine. Many of her problems centered around dates with boys and doing the right thing by her parents, authority figures, and friends.

2. Sullivan defines chumship as "the intimate exchange of empathy which permits the capacity of seeing one's self through the other's eyes" (p. 261). Sullivan thought chumship was particularly important during preadolescence.

group. Later, an art-therapy workshop was added. I supervised all groups.

The group leaders carefully assisted the formation of peer relationships. Patients in groups were able to experience new forms of relating and to confront aspects of self-experience from which they dissociated. I purposefully remained in the background to absorb the more difficult transference reactions and to give patients room to move freely and to determine for themselves how close they wanted to bring themselves to psychological observation.

When a difficulty in a friendship pair or unit emerged, couples counseling was made available. Couples counseling functioned as a forum for learning how to be in a relationship. This protocol was also elaborated into a series of "dating workshops" to offer guidance in the formation of significant-other pairings.

Confronting Reality Issues

All participants in the program were asked to participate in a six-part course. The first two classes were about medical aspects of HIV and AIDS. Medical secrets became shared knowledge. Current information was provided so that patients could more positively interact with their doctors.

The next class was about safe sex, with a colorful presentation that accentuated the realities of their lifestyle. A transvestite member of the class taught everybody how to place a condom on a man who refuses to wear one while performing oral sex. A fourth class on human intimacy addressed the emotional side of sexuality, something that had remained obscure to them. Later, a nutritionist, dentist, and ophthalmologist offered classes too.

The class made it acceptable to think, to question, to learn, to know, and thereby to transcend limitations that they imposed on themselves and that others reinforced. I added a corollary program to assist people in obtaining their high school diplomas, and to support people who wanted to learn to read or to go to college.

I started a spirituality group to address sociocultural issues and to discuss the patients' experiences of injustice. It was one thing to experience one's self as liminal, yet another to be liminal and poor; but to be liminal, poor, and dying added new proportions to the term "hopeless." I taught them about Abraham Joshua Heschel, a rabbi and Jewish philosopher who worked closely with Martin Luther King, and about liberation theology. The concept of cultural and historical processes beyond their own, I believed, could induce curiosity and establish an observational perspective that provided distance from the intense affect states accompanying fears of death. The observational stance could lessen self-deprecating feelings and suggest less self-condemnatory explanations for their life histories. A more balanced sense of self would enable my deeply frightened patients to choose self-expression over self-destructive behavior as a coping mechanism.

We read aloud because some patients couldn't read. Our first readings were from Heschel (1963) and included "The Patient as a Person." Discussing God, the doctor-patient relationship, and the feelings of liminality stimulated an awareness that their personal problems existed at a more global level. They realized that the world is as troubled a place as their own lives. The group became important for the generation of hope as some of their difficult social circumstances were validated. I acknowledged with them that racism, sexism, classism, and homophobia exist. As my patients felt more secure about the accuracy of their perceptions, I was able to work with them on the more threatening question—Now What?

As their reality was confirmed, it was easier to address and set limits on behaviors that were unhealthy toward self and others. Working honestly and reflectively with their maladaptive behavior necessitated that I confront the prejudices that caused me to lower my expectations to accommodate to a person's deprived background. They, in turn, had to confront their own self-prejudices so as not to similarly rationalize their antisocial activity. In this way, we could get to work on the psychological issues underlying HIV and AIDS.

Integration

Once the group program and friendship patterns were established, I became motivated to push the people with whom I worked to integrate their strengths and weaknesses. Active members of the group program were invited to become peer counselors, because one way to get some people to become patients was to make them doctors. I taught them what I knew about psychology, psychoanalysis, and HIV disease.

Members of this program became angry when I didn't work hard enough to keep attendance in the program high. They criticized me when I failed to create new projects. They were disappointed by the delays in purchasing a coffee pot and new furniture. I explained that if I did all the work for the program, I would get all the credit. Although parts of me enjoyed "the good doctor" role, all that would be left for them was work associated to "the patient role."

They became willing to exchange their dependent roles—and all the bad self-associations they had to such a role—for active roles that utilized their personal strengths and potentials. They made curtains for the group room, planned workshops and events, and became group leaders and individual counselors. In challenging their idealization of me, I asked to be more human. I relied on the durability of our interactions to establish a therapeutic frame, and not on the consummate fantasies often projected onto the role of psychologist.

Adaptations of Psychotherapy

While working in the group program, patients had the chance to develop the degree of trust necessary for individual psychotherapy. I had to accommodate the process, however, to the demands of a difficult patient population, to the needs of someone who was not yet acutely ill, and to those of someone who would soon die. I changed the way I worked. The nature of the changes assumed three forms.

Adaptations to a Difficult Patient Population

In an effort to make sense of a difficult caseload, I organized my patients according to their process style. I grouped my patients into three loose categories that were based on their interactive style with me: the far, the proximal, and the close.

Patients who use far discourse, quite naturally, experience therapy from a distance. They regularly schedule appointments they don't keep. In this way, they keep themselves in my mind, and me in theirs. In lieu of actual sessions, they engage me in the hall, outside the hospital, or occasionally in the neighborhood, for "brief therapeutic encounters." They often act as though we have an important connection, even though I struggle to remember them. Some people who relate in this manner eventually become interested in, and tolerant of, more extensive treatment. Even within the far-discourse mode of relating, however, many derive benefits.

Jacinto, a 25-year-old Hispanic male, was an excellent example of somebody who was comfortable with far discourse. He never kept an appointment, but he made a new one every time he saw me. During these encounters he rapidly updated me on the progress of his life. Before I could respond he would say something like, "I know what you are trying to tell me. You think I'm not dealing with my underlying issues. I know I need to work on why I'm stopping myself from getting a better life." In this fashion, he stopped using drugs, remained out of jail, discontinued a destructive relationship, and was accepted into college. Although I never had a session with this man, he always referred to me as his psychologist. A full therapy session may have been over-stimulating. I had to respect his titration of our relationship.

People who engage at the proximal level actually come for regular sessions, but they find it difficult to speak and use the experience. My work with them focuses on concrete objectives. I also nurture curiosity and create a safe and helpful environment for self-expression.

For instance, Michael, a 42-year-old African-American man—"the man of many Dalmatians," as he called himself—was suspicious and paranoid of "the system." Initially he wouldn't talk in session and would only stay for a few minutes. He later began to quiz me, and he wondered if I was trying to figure him out. I told him I was curious but that he had me stumped. I didn't have a clue as to what was going on with him. His twice-weekly psychotherapy sessions lengthened and we played word games. We "chatted." During the course of our talking, we began to agree or disagree on which words we could use to describe the topic of our conversation. When he described "the man who becomes others" (his term), I acknowledged the person as "the man with blond hair." He explained, "His hair isn't really blond." I agreed. I said it might have had some brown in it. This continued until we had arrived at a mutually acceptable way of discussing the color of this man's hair, "Brownish blond with a bit of auburn at the roots." Our relationship evolved from the hybrid language we created together.

Leroy, a 43-year-old African-American man, was another person who took a proximal approach to therapy. He was on parole, a drug addict, and a recent convert to Islam. He struck me as polite, sincere, and well-mannered. He always called me "Ma'am." I wondered aloud with him how it was possible that he had done all the awful things he described to me. He wanted to know the same thing. He explained, "It's just that when I use drugs, I'm not me. It's just a not-me experience."

Not knowing how close his use of the term was to Sullivan's (1953), I nonetheless pulled out a piece of drawing paper and asked my patient to draw me his "not-me" self. Then I asked for his "good-me" and "bad-me" selves. He then listed behaviors that fell under each category. Under "not-me" he included everything he did while on drugs: criminal, manipulative, and sexually exploitative behavior. He listed under "bad-me" his skin color, failing to protect his nieces from incest, disappointing his parents, and not learning to read. "Good-me" included his family loyalty, caretaking abilities, and sensitivity. He used to care for hurt animals, help an elderly woman in his building, and feed hungry people.

Two months later, he was admitted to another hospital with a severe PCP and inflammation of the brain. I suspected tubercular meningitis. He called me to let me know that he had figured out that all the selves were really "all him." He said, "I'm the all-me self." He died shortly thereafter. I was happy that he had discovered some inkling of reconciliation with himself.

My last example of proximal therapy was our star patient, Howard. Howard was a recently paroled 34-year-old white male. He confessed that he had killed an infant when he burned down the home of a drug foe and served time for murder. All his problems, he explained, were due to a horrendous drug problem. Within months, he had completely given up drugs, obtained benefits, and entered a job-training program. He was about to leave the shelter in which he had been living to get his own apartment. A series of chance encounters revealed that the parole department had no record of him. He had not applied for any benefits. There was no job-training program. Because he had no physical evidence of a drug habit and, in fact, no test for HIV, it became apparent that this man was deeply involved in a fantasy about himself. Attempts to confront him provoked painful excuses and rationalizations. We agreed to keep treating him on the grounds that we couldn't determine that he didn't have HIV disease. I saw him therapeutically for almost a year after our discovery. I continued to work with the person he believed himself to be, and he was still being treated for HIV disease. During one session, he said with a telling wink, "Don't be surprised if I turn out differently than you expected." I told him he already had.

Close discourse is what we more typically think of as therapy. I only saw about eight patients in this manner, some of whom were initially far-discourse patients. Sessions with people who can work in close-discourse mode nicely reflect how HIV and AIDS issues interacted with psychodynamic issues.

Stephen was a 40-year-old musician of mixed ethnicity—Asian and French—who had solved his substance-abuse problems over the past five years. He was raised by maternal grandparents who felt responsible for their daughter's failed life. She was a substance abuser. Stephen burdened and overwhelmed them. He recognized that he wasted his life on "needing, pleasing, and teasing others" to fill a "deep insecurity and sadness," the belief that he was worthless. While discussing a recent performance, he stated, "the pressure is fantastic."

I asked him to describe the pressure and he associated his "performance anxiety" to needing to "help Betty" (a fellow group member who was dying). He described how hard it was to watch her deteriorate, and expressed a need to change his life before it was too late.

He said, "I feel like I'm hurriedly flipping though a pile of index cards looking for the answers."

I asked what was on the cards. He explained he was rushing by them too fast and that he had no time to stop and read them. We agreed that if he had the cards, he must already have some answers.

He blurted out, "But I want to get there now. I am a man dying before his time. I will be dead within a year and all I want to know is that I mattered and that I count and that my life has been about something." He paused, then continued, "I need to save someone. And if I can't save Betty, and I can't save myself, and I never saved my mother. . . ."

He cried. He connected feeling worthless to never having been able to help anybody. He decided that as long as he was alive he wanted to be effective and useful. He wanted to die as a person who mattered. He needed to know that something he had done was good enough to have helped someone.

Adaptations to Patients with Extended Life Spans

When people are diagnosed HIV-positive, they often experience a period of dramatic intensity and crisis. They are eager to change and want to push themselves to work on the issues of their lives. However, once it becomes clear that they aren't acutely ill and won't be dying anytime soon they often retreat to a more relaxed process.

It is intolerable and inhumane to require someone always to keep his illness in mind. A degree of denial is effective, adaptive, and necessary. As a therapist, I respect a person's boundaries. Yet, I don't collude with defensive processes. I walk the tightrope between confrontation and passivity. It is difficult to know where to stand, and I use questions to find a comfortable balance. I ask if something that is happening is related to the experience of being HIV-positive. I share that it was hard to know what can be discussed. I request that I be told how and when to get close.

A second and related issue is that a psychologist working with HIV-positive persons is often associated with "death." This disrupts therapeutic continuity. If patients want to avoid issues of death they simply avoid the therapist. One patient told me, "Every time I come to session I feel like I'm going to choose which coffin I should be buried in. If I don't come, I don't ever have to make that choice." Instead, we worked together to establish a relationship that gave him room to flee and to remain heavily engaged in life. Making new friends, seeking new relationships, and pursuing goals were as important as verbalizing the fear of dying.

The third thing I developed was an ability to remain calm and not overreact to dramatic dynamics. On a given day, some people might weep uncontrollably, scream vehemently, and reveal psychotic-like processes. Persons with HIV need a safe place for these very primary emotions, yet they also need careful limits because they might otherwise lose the real people in their lives who can't contain or deal with what those intense feelings provoke in them.

Finally, issues of diagnosis are troubling and difficult because the stress of death tends to exaggerate underlying symptoms and character pathology. Although I worked within established diagnostic categories, I paid more attention to how people used or didn't use relationships. This was a better diagnostic and prognostic indicator.

Adaptations When Someone Is Close to Death

When someone is close to death, there are no useful generalities. Every death is unique to the dying person and the people he or she leaves behind. People with AIDS die in stages, often losing one aspect of themselves at a time. For instance, John was a well-loved man who had been a performer most of his life. He developed HIV dementia long before he was sick with a major opportunistic infection. He couldn't remember names, the date, or the time, but every time I came to his room, he smiled. It was the part of his personality that remained. He clung to it with a fervor that at times shamed me.

Ray was a 45-year-old black man who lived most of his life in a single residence occupancy hotel. He had a heroin addiction for more than 20 years. His only family member came to the hospital to pick up his checks and didn't stop to visit. I liked Ray. I respected his honesty about who he was. Fascinated by his kindness and his unwillingness to blame anyone for his addictions or other problems, I enjoyed listening to his life story. He saw life from the bottom up, and his perspective interested me because he challenged my liberalism. I wanted to help. He asked only for my company and the chance to tell his story. His physical condition deteriorated. Finally he could only listen to the radio while he clutched my hand. I remembered that he was a jazz fan, so I arranged for a semi-well-known musician to come play saxophone for him. The musician played for hours while my friend Ray wept. He died two days later while trying to stand up.

I worked with Betty, a 32-year-old African-American woman. I met her mother and her brother. She was raised in a strict home where both her parents lived until her father's death almost 15 years ago. He worked in a factory all day. At night, at home, he worked the bottle. He had been an alcoholic all her early life. Betty loved his charm, his humor, and his musicality. She resented her mother's uptight ways. As she grew up, Betty experimented with alcohol, then with drugs. Her father died when she was in her early 20s. Her drug use escalated. Her mother changed the locks on the doors. She slept in the subways. It was her HIV diagnosis that convinced her to seek recovery.

By the time I met her, she had been off drugs for three years. She became one of the first peer counselors in the program. Energetic, savvy, and soulful, Betty's presence was an instrumental force in the group program. Sometimes her groups had as many as 30 people in them. Many referred to her as their inspiration. She witnessed that she touched people. Finally she was living a life of which her father would have been proud. She was reluctant to try therapy. She explained, "It will make it too hard for me to leave. Let's do this from a distance." I followed her wishes. Our work together concentrated on her training as a group leader.

No one anticipated that she would become ill with opportunistic infections as quickly as she did. A mere seven months after being diagnosed with fibroid tumors and other gynecological infections, she lay wasting away in her hospital bed with a rapid onset dementia. The people in the program organized a vigil. Someone sat by her side at all possible times. Another group of people took care of her mother and siblings. They made food deliveries to their home and supported them, too. My job was to support her friends, her fellow group members, so that they could tolerate accompanying her to death. Her work in the group program fulfilled her dream of who she might have been without drugs. Sitting at the center of a group of 25 people and eliciting from them deep emotions about their difficult struggles with drugs was the most important achievement in her life. My role as her psychologist was to protect the growth she had achieved in this last part of her life. She died a group leader, and not an addict.

James, a 42-year-old African-American male, was in the program for 10 months. A converted Muslim and former drug addict, he learned to play guitar and write poetry and became the loading-dock foreman at his job before AIDS caught up with him. He was curious about psychoanalysis and wanted to work intensely. Soon into our work, he became very ill with aspergillosis of the lung. Physical limitations precluded talking very much together. We watched Oprah Winfrey together on the TV in his hospital room. Blind, and in renal and liver failure, literally hours before he died, he told me, in a soft and quivering voice, that I was the only white person, much less white woman, that he had ever known. Our relationship had made him rethink race. White people weren't so bad, and maybe color was a more complicated issue than he had realized. He was glad for the knowledge. He had something to show God.

Conclusion

I have found that the people I have worked with at the hospital needed me to respect them. I grappled with the limits of their humanity by being honest about my own. In so doing, I have learned to live better and have been influenced by what my patients taught me. The depth at which people work when ill enabled me to observe personality in some of its most undisguised manifestations. In some cases, I was the only person who knew the real story of someone's life. I have seen the best and the worst of people. I have found the middle ground in the territory between self and other known as *relationship*. This motivated me to invest in my work and my life. I resolved my anguish about other people's unfulfilled potential by becoming eager and determined about my own.

Jenny, a 38-year-old white female, and I have worked together since my first day at the hospital when she threw up at my feet. Nervous and apologetic, she explained her crack problem. I recognized an anger in her gesture, and a statement about authority. Her irreverence summoned my courage to work with her. Over the years, Jenny has let me know when and how people, including me, have violated her boundaries. She has screamed in my office. She has attacked herself.

We have confronted competition in our relationship. I found myself fantasizing that I was a better mother to her than her own mother. The fantasy perpetuated Jenny's tendency to split her world into strict good or bad polarities. As the "good" or "superior" psychologist, I patronized her "bad" mother, and thereby the "bad" Jenny. To work together in a more equal fashion has required that I search my personality for remnants of the traits that could have made me a crack addict. Jenny explained, "Don't keep me down by acting as if this could never happen to you."

I answered her, "I can imagine this happening to me, and that is important. But it hasn't. We have to find some way of relating together that feels equal and doesn't deny our differences." So we have constructed a relationship that confronts the very difficult issues of what unites and separates people. There has been constant motion between us. We have tried to build a relationship that isn't based on who is on top and who is on the bottom. We have acknowledged real status and health differences. The interplay between us is dialectical. Its resolution has been seen in Jenny's four years without drugs. She has lived in and maintained her own apartment. She has enrolled in college. She has volunteered for many agencies and organizations. She began her first part-time job. Jenny said, "I have to keep thinking of what I can still be . . . I have to use hope like a mirror."

We, patients and psychologist, influenced and changed one another. I have remembered the personality traits and life stories of dying people. This has pushed my own development. I don't doubt that seeking analytic training and opening a private practice, instead of settling into life as an institutional psychologist, was fueled by my patients' wishes that they could have fulfilled similar dreams. They passed that opportunity on to me. Life's chances were easily discernible from the death bed. No one wished to remain stagnant. My commitment to growth has been my tribute to the people I have known and lost. The only way to transcend survivor's guilt is to have survived.

Ever since my teens, I have always wanted to be the philosopher and social scientist Hannah Arendt. Instead, I became a Gidget. The people in the group program didn't need a Hannah. They needed a Gidget, and it was by accepting her at her best that I discovered the basic honesty and integrity of therapeutic work.

References

Geertz, C. (1973), *The Interpretation of Cultures.* New York: Basic Books.

Heschel, A. J. (1965), *Who is Man?* Stanford, CA: Stanford University Press.

Hillman, J. (1996), *The Soul's Code.* New York: Random House.

Sullivan, H. S. (1953), *The Interpersonal Theory of Psychiatry.* New York: Norton.

Turner, V. (1969), *The Ritual Process.* Ithaca, NY: Cornell University Press.

Part 2
CASE STUDIES

5 There but for the Grace of . . .

Countertransference During the Psychotherapy of a Young HIV-Positive Woman

Sue A. Shapiro

I sit down to write and find that I have no thoughts, no theories, no meaning. *This* is my countertransference. It's quite unlike me. It parallels J's difficulty in settling on a meaning for her life, settling on a direction, a career path.

What is a legitimate form for this chapter to take? There's no single story to tell, no single formulation to make sense of it all. For the purposes of this book, J's story is that of the psychoanalytically informed treatment of an HIV-positive woman from an upper-middle-class family who has shunned traditional medicine and has opted instead for a variety of alternative treatments. But J is also a child of divorce, a child of 60s parents who have been through their share of drugs, alcohol, sex, changes in values, and changes in financial status over time. She is also a former child actress-performer. Hers is the story of adolescent rebellion, including drugs, self-mutilation, and an attraction to life in the streets. It is the story of someone who does not have to work to survive. And it is a story of sexual freedom and experimentation with men and women, richly varied, and of "growing up," settling down, straightening. It is the story of a passage from adolescence to adulthood, a passage shaped by AIDS.

Becoming HIV-positive alters meaning, alters time. Treating someone who has this diagnosis likewise changes my sense of purpose and meaning. They say life is a fatal illness. But most of the time, most of the people I see in my practice keep intimations of mortality far, far away. One woman went so far as to be highly insulted when I challenged her use of the conditional phrase "if my parents ever die." "If?" I asked. What do you mean? You mean "when," don't you? "No! If," she insisted. Such denial of death is not limited to patients or young people. So this story, my work with J over the last seven years, during long stretches of which we were separated by a continent, is also the story of two people addressing their mortality, separately and together.

J was referred to me two years after my mother died following a heroic struggle with cancer. She died on July 15, 1987, one week after the sudden death of my uncle, one day before a fatal aneurysm killed my stepgrandfather, and one week before another uncle's heart gave out. This two-week period was the culmination of a two-year period in my life marked by death—eight deaths, to be exact. Some were sudden, like my father's from a car accident, or his brother's from a massive coronary; some were like my mother's, expected after long illness. Some deaths came at the end of long lives—men and women in their 80s and 90s—other deaths cut short the still-vigorous lives of people in their 50s and 60s.

My life was forever changed by these events. My sense of meaning, purpose, duration, time, community, and permanence would never be the same. I had come from a very long-lived family. I watched my grandmother at 75 tend to her mother when she died at 97. This is what I expected would be my story as well. I was wrong.

I was still in the midst of mourning when I was asked if I could work with J, a young woman who had recently found out she was HIV-positive. The referring therapist thought I'd be uniquely suited to work with J because of my own history. The styles and interests of our families of origin overlapped considerably. We both grew up in Manhattan, both experienced our parents' divorce at a young age, both came from musical families, both were into alternative treatments, and both were quite rebellious in our teens and 20s. But there were some critical differences: I was 16 years older. My parents were products of the 40s and 50s; hers were products of the 60s. I came of age in the 60s and early 70s, she in the late 70s and 80s.

I was in Haight Ashbury in the summer of love and had my first macrobiotic meal when coming down from my first acid trip in 1968. There was plenty of sex in those days of newly discovered freedom. There were some risks: abortion was still illegal, and I remember taking up a collection in college for a friend to go to Mexico for an illegal abortion. We were all on the pill, although we had to endure the moralizing speeches of the gynecologists who ambivalently prescribed them. Condoms were a thing of the past. There were, of course, STDs (we didn't have that acronym yet), the old fashioned ones, gonorrhea and syphilis, during that brief moment in time when everything seemed curable.

All my friends experimented with drugs. Few of us drank and I didn't know anyone who I thought got hooked on anything. There were a couple of casualties from bad acid trips. There were also some people I thought were tripping, but I later found out that they hadn't taken anything at all and never stopped "tripping." There was no cocaine that I knew of in college, but there was plenty of speed—how else could papers get written? There were people rumored to shoot up heroin—they were really cool. In fact, I went out with two of them. One eventually cleaned up his act, got a Ph.D. in molecular biology, and then died in a mountaineering accident. The other stopped using heroin, went on to travel, live in Japan, marry a Japanese woman, move back, have a baby, write a novel, and become HIV-positive in the early 1990s.

And me? I survived the 60s, I don't remember them well (you see, I really *was* there). In September 1969, after a year in San Francisco, I came back East for graduate school and my gradual "straightening." My time out West left me with an enduring interest in yoga, health food, macrobiotics, alternative medicine, and body work. I also chose to live and work downtown, in "The Village."

For these reasons, it looked like I would be a good match for J.

J was referred to me a year or two into her own "straightening." She had returned from the West Coast to audition for a major Broadway musical. She just missed getting the role, became depressed, started therapy, and decided to clean up her act. She stopped using heroin, worked for a while as a staff person in a detox program, ended her relationship with her Latino lover, who also abused drugs, and decided to get tested for HIV. J tested positive in May 1987 and believes she seroconverted back in 1984 in Paris. Two years later, one of J's best friends also tested positive—she too had been in Paris. Around the time that J discovered she was positive, her stepbrother was diagnosed with a malignant brain tumor. He died one year later, at the age of 16.

During the late 70s and early 80s J used a variety of drugs. Some she got turned on to by her father, others she found on her own—downtown, on the street, where "things seemed true," unlike the hypocrisy she felt at home. Although the drive to abuse drugs came from a complex and conflicted childhood, there was also a craving for new and more intense experiences, and there was the sheer hedonism of the time and place: New York City, and specifically the East Village. We were later to discover, as well, an ongoing search for meaning, for altered states, for a spiritual dimension to life, a search that crisscrossed her life from very early on. During these years there was both casual and committed sex with men and women, time spent in school, in acting and performance work, and in odd jobs, such as waitressing and go-go dancing in lesbian bars by which she supported herself. J had a fascination with black and Hispanic culture, the culture of the kids in her neighborhood who alternately taunted her and welcomed her.

I knew from the referring therapist that at the time of the referral, J was involved with a "nice" man, someone who was in recovery himself, someone whom her family approved of and hoped she would marry. They had met after she discovered her HIV status and were currently living together. I remember wondering and asking the referring therapist, "Is he positive too?" "No." "Does he know?" "Yes." I didn't voice my next thought, the obvious: "And still they are together?" My prejudices and preconceptions were all there. I still hadn't met her. I sensed some pressure to get her married. I wondered what kind of guy her boyfriend Paul was.

As I write this, I remember something I've forgotten for the last several years, but which was deeply resonant during that first, referring phone call: my father's second marriage to Dorothy, a 28-year-old woman with Hodgkin's disease. I remember my father explaining to me, as an adult, the conversation he had had with Dorothy's parents after he found this out.

"How could you not tell me she has Hodgkin's disease? I've just been through a messy divorce and so has my seven-year-old daughter!"

"We want our daughter to have a normal life," they said. "She doesn't know she's terminally ill. She's 28 and we just want her to be happy."

My father struggled with his decision. He loved Dorothy, wanted to be with her, and he eventually decided to go ahead with the wedding. But several times his anxiety and ambivalence got the better of him, and the wedding was postponed because of his physical illnesses. Finally they married. Nine months later she was dead. But this deed was recalled when my father was eulogized, and in my memory it remains the best thing he ever did. It is probably also significant that I credit Dorothy with being a very positive influence in my life and saw her as a gentle, nonjudgmental alternative to my highly critical and demanding parents.

From this perspective I wondered about Paul, J's boyfriend. I wondered what kind of man he was, and I wondered what lay in store for him and for them as a couple. I wondered whether or not his family knew and whether or not they approved. I also wondered what lay in store for me if J and I chose to work together.

Until this moment in 1989, I had not treated anyone who I knew was HIV-positive, although I had treated several people with multiple losses due to AIDS. I had lost only acquaintances through this disease, no one I was deeply committed to, no one I had seen through this process.

J came into my office for the first time, unaware of the layers of feeling, memory, and fantasy already present in me. She was young, pretty: wild black hair, long dreadlocks—are they real? Tiny, thin, articulate, determined, opinionated. There's something about her I like a lot, but I sense she won't be easy to reach.

J didn't at first say anything about being HIV-positive, and somewhere in those first fumbling minutes I let on that I knew. "What? He told you I was HIV-positive? I didn't say he could do that." We were off to an awkward start. But I think my office decor, which included Tibetan tankas and lots of rocks and crystals, and my generally informal style helped buy me some time. I think she and I sat on the floor that day, but maybe I just felt that's where we should have been. The meeting continued.

"I can't choose a career, I don't know whether to be a singer or not. It's all tied up with my mother—she's a song writer, and my father—he's a musician.

"I sang for my family. I sang the blues and the grownups thought it was amazing that I had this sexy voice. I don't know what style to sing in—my mother says this, the music industry wants that, none of it is me. I hate the music industry people— they're sleazy, unhealthy. The clubs are filled with smoke and the shows start at 11 at night, about when I should be getting to bed."

How much can I, or should I, ask about her health? Her T cells? What's she doing about her health? Safe sex? Will I alienate her if I ask all this too soon, or is it irresponsible if I wait? I choose to wait, sensing that much of this is my anxiety.

"I gave Paul a vial of my blood. It's the one thing we can't share."

I'm sure that's not the way we started to talk about being positive, but she told me this in one of our first sessions.

I think we began to speak about HIV because J and Paul were trying to decide about a trip to Africa. It looked like Paul would have some work there and J really wanted to go. Her parents were trying to dissuade her.

"What's your policy about missed sessions? My last therapist expected me to pay, but I don't know, I want to travel."

Well, there we were, right in our first session, in the midst of central issues. What is J's voice, what is her calling? And how important is regular structure? We were about to start therapy, and already there was this talk of breaks and long trips—not generally a good sign. But what makes sense for a young woman who doesn't know how long she has to live? Do you invest in the long term? Do you live for today? Do I serve her best by trying to conduct a treatment by the rules, thereby conveying faith in her ongoing living? Am I conveying my pessimism if I change the rules? Can I honestly say therapy is more important than travel, than living to the max, having experiences while it is still possible? These questions, in one form or another, are often in the room with us during our work together.

And then there are the more expectable treatment issues: What is J's "style"? What is her "voice"? How can she separate from her parents without denying or killing off the talents they recognize and appreciate? How much of life must be determined by whether or not it is healthful? These were the central questions that would continue to inform our work over the next seven years.

These questions are really not so different from the questions that inform many treatments: who am I, where am I going, what is the meaning of it all? I often wonder what J would be like, what the work with her would have been like, if she had not seroconverted. In many ways, the issues that we struggle with are the issues that affect many educated, upper-middle-class, talented young women in the years between age 26 and 33. What kind of career shall I have? Do I want to invest years in learning a skill that I may or may not enjoy using? Can I get started right away? Must I express myself with my native talents? Do I owe it to my friends, family, the world? How ambitious am I? What is of central importance, what gives my life meaning? Should I get into a committed relationship? Where should I live? Should I have children? Do I have to give up sex with other people? But with J, all of these issues were explored through this thick surround of imminent illness. At times we would almost forget its presence, and then fatigue, a cold, or an especially vivid dream would bring us back to that reality. It never really left us.

Africa was deemed too dangerous. In fact, many of her longed-for destinations in Asia and Africa were off limits, given the risks of disease and the risks from prophylaxis—the vaccines or the antimalarial medications. I breathed a sigh of relief when J made this decision and was able to forgo immediate pleasure in making her choice. Deciding against this trip also allowed us to get started, and it really took some time for us to check each other out and find our way together. J feared my prejudices against her former lifestyle and life choices and about her current health state. I feared being irresponsible through ignorance, getting close and being abandoned, and too, I feared contagion. I knew this was irrational, but I couldn't help hesitating before I sat down on the toilet after J was in the bathroom, or wondering how carefully I needed to wash a cup she drank from. Fortunately, during this time I could consult with Mark Blechner who had worked with many AIDS patients and was writing on the subject. He could both normalize my fears and underscore their irrationality.

But then there were gray areas—there still are. Do I call J when I have a cold and give her the option of canceling? When the weather is terrible and I know she has a long way to go, is it better if she comes or stays home? How careful do she and Paul have to be about sex? How much of this is my business? At what point do I sit back with some comfort, knowing they are making informed decisions, taking informed risks? And lately, there is the question of children.

It took at least a year for me to realize that J was not at all in denial, that she was generally very responsible in taking care of her medical needs and in her concern for others. Over time, I learned how she had contacted all her past lovers after finding out she was positive and how relieved she was that all of them were negative. I learned of her initial fears of being undesirable and of how some men and women chose not to have sex with her when they knew her HIV status. I learned about her friends' reactions, of J's resilience and her ability to start new relationships, including sexual ones.

Paul and J decided to take part in a study of heterosexual couples in which one member was HIV-positive. J felt that participation in this study gave her no new information, and she and Paul disliked the cold, clinical atmosphere. But I was relieved knowing that they were being monitored and getting ongoing information from people I viewed as experts about the relative safety of various sex acts. For some time now they haven't had sex during J's period, they use condoms for intercourse, and they enjoy unprotected oral sex.

When I first met J, her T cells had been declining, but she was otherwise symptom free. Well—not exactly. Two health areas had been ongoing problems throughout J's life: upper respiratory infections and vaginal candida. During those first years of work together it dawned on us that she was almost always slightly ill. J had been seeing a Western doctor known for his holistic treatments. I think it was the endless yeast infections that started J on her quest for new treatments, something beyond the vitamin drips she was already receiving. First there was the anticandida diet: no sugar, no alcohol, no wheat, no caffeine, no fermented products. This was the beginning of an ongoing journey through various alternative treatments, diets, and healers. At some point there was the first visit to a psychic, then a new nutritionist, an astrologer, and so on. Getting off sugar was bad; it was like getting off drugs, she said. Days of aimlessness, groggy, fuzzy-headed, craving sugar, craving something, unable to concentrate. New words were used to describe and explain sensations and symptoms: "It's the 'die off,' that is why you feel worse when you start to cleanse your body. First you feel terrible, then you feel much better." Gradually an alternative treatment team was falling into place. Increasingly in therapy there were discussions of family history, career choices, friendships, her relationship with Paul, and eventually our relationship as well. At times I felt competitive with, and envious of, the other members of J's treatment team. The psychic, Andrea, and various other people J consulted could give specific, although often cryptic, advice and information. I felt, and our therapy felt, so mundane. There were several crises in which J felt our work wasn't going deep enough or fast enough. At times these alerted us to specific irritations and disappointments with me, ways that I was perhaps coddling her, not being confrontational enough. At other times they reflected J's general frustrations, disappointments, craving for intensity, and sense of urgency.

I was familiar with some of the diets and treatments that J tried; they interested me independently of her. I often would try these diets to see what she was experiencing. When she was feeling well, J would start to worry about her career. She would start singing lessons or work up a demo tape, and arrange some local performances. Singing remained conflict-laden. Performing was something she had to do for her mother's friends, but also something she loved to do. Her friends and family felt she had to sing—it was too great a gift to turn her back on. But for J, singing not only meant ties to her family but ties to an unhealthy lifestyle of cigarettes, drugs, and sexual innuendo. The songs she loved to sing were the blues. They came from sadness and pain, but they also pushed her voice in unhealthy ways. J couldn't imagine singing the trivial lyrics of many contemporary songs, and she couldn't imagine writing songs when she was happy or in a stable relationship—when she wasn't heartsick. But now she was planning a wedding.

J's wedding, like most weddings, was a compromise. The ceremony and location were partially a compromise, and the decision to marry represented a compromise. Paul was sweet, loving, gentle, reliable, and at times romantic, but he wasn't intense and dangerous. Paul was in recovery but had never been in therapy, and he was not engaged in deep self-exploration. "He's not in touch with his feelings," J would complain. And I would think, "What will he do if he gets more in touch with his feelings? Maybe this is the only way he can go ahead and get married." For a long time I feared saying this to J, and I don't know if we spoke of it before the wedding. But we have been able to discuss this and over time Paul has become more expressive and emotional.

Informing the prewedding tension was the secret of J's HIV status. At the time of the wedding, Paul's family didn't know. It wasn't until several years later, as an outgrowth of their first couple-therapy session, that J and Paul began to tell them.

I don't often go to patients' weddings, but in this case I decided to—in part because of the weight of secrecy and also because, by now, I loved J and wanted to share in this moment. I was glad to be there, to meet her family and exchange a knowing look, to see her friends, and to see her and Paul as joyous as a couple can be.

The years and themes blend. By December 1990, when I needed to go in for minor surgery, J was already deeply immersed in the work of Susan Weed, author of *Healing Wise,* an important book on herbal remedies. J recommended various alternatives to surgery. I was already committed to having the surgery but decided to try some of these methods as well. I was struck by how labor-intensive they are, how active I had to be in my own healing, and how much faith I would have needed to pursue this way to the exclusion of more drastic, Western, fighting ways.

The more J pursued alternative treatments, the more all-consuming they became—the more they affected her whole life. She was committed to living healthfully. Would it be possible to do this and pursue a career? It was difficult enough just having a job. Much of what our culture expects from people as a sign of their commitment to their careers—a sign of their ambitiousness—is deeply at odds with a healthy lifestyle. Many of us are aware of this, many of our patients complain about it, but for J this posed an urgent problem. Periodically J would get a job, but her old ways of supporting herself through waitressing or work in a club no longer seemed worth the price she paid with her health. Smoked-filled rooms and nighttime hours wore her down. At times J would get interesting work, related to a possible career, but it would require working 12- and 15-hour days. She then wouldn't eat as well, wouldn't exercise, and her health would suffer. Not having a career, especially when her husband was working long hours, left J feeling peripheral, uncentered, and weak, as though her life completely revolved around Paul's.

The conflicts between J and her family began to be enacted around health issues. Her mother and stepfather smoked heavily and, in J's opinion, drank excessively. But J was also quite close to her mother and was grateful as well for the financial support she received during these last years. The support enabled her to pursue treatments, travel occasionally, and take lessons and courses. But this support, and the parents' concern about her well-being, coexist, in J's opinion, with an expressed denial of, and indifference to, J's physical concerns and needs. Literally, her mother's house was toxic—J got physically ill after spending time there. J learned to speak up to friends and family to protect herself. This speaking up seemed necessary for both her physical and emotional health.

Increasingly, J's life centered around being HIV-positive and healing herself and others. J often said that she had always felt there was something wrong with her, and HIV became a ready container for feelings she had had all her life—feelings that arose in response to her parent's divorce when she was two, the sense of estrangement she experienced when her stepfather moved in, her learning difficulties, her precocious sexuality. Andrea, the psychic, told J early on that she had to read about the Persephone myth and had to make a difficult but necessary journey to the underworld. J's journey into being HIV-positive, learning to face her fears and keep herself healthy, has also been her journey into exploring her sense of badness and her confusion surrounding her identity (her class, her work, J the temptress, J the priestess). This journey is powerfully expressed in songs that she has written over the last year and a half.

Her earlier identity confusion expressed itself in the first years of treatment in clothing and "packing" dreams. In these dreams, J was forever packing and trying to decide what outfits to bring, or coming up with elaborate costumes to wear. She had had dreams like this all her life. I heard them in terms of J's background of early divorcing parents, her lifelong fascination with clothing and costumes, an emphasis on appearances in lieu of something deeper—a need to dress the part in order, hopefully, to inhabit the role. I also felt that her experienced and expressed anxiety over packing helped delay the terrifying trip.

In the first years of treatment, this dream-theme of identity confusion alternated with very dramatic HIV dreams in which themes of infection, premature death, separation, and difference from others predominated. These dreams return whenever J is especially worried about her health. But they became less frequent as J found other ways of expressing her fears. She began to keep a journal, and in her singing class she began to sing of AIDS—not with words but with sounds. At a women's healing weekend, J stunned her group during the final hours with a long, wordless, spontaneous spiritual. She also began to think about making a movie.

Alongside this increased creativity, J began to give herbal advice to friends. She learned some hands-on healing techniques, and found she was quite talented at this, quite skilled in working with people's bodies and energy. But the emotional and physical toll of this form of healing work seemed too great, she became too exhausted. J began to think that verbal psychotherapy would be a safer way of working with people.

J considered applying to social-work school, where she expected to learn theories of treatment as well as ways of protecting herself from the debilitating immersion in other people to which she was prone. But school would take time, would require working in hospitals and exposing herself to infection, and would mean spending several years preparing to start a new life. It also meant spending several uninterrupted years in New York.

By this time in our work, J had developed a pattern of leaving the city for one or two months in the winter and at least one in the summer. Her health always improved when she was in simple, warmer surroundings. Also, Paul's work was sporadic and often involved moving to another part of the country for several months. J didn't want a prolonged absence from him and felt that because he had a career and she didn't, she should follow him. This left J feeling uncentered, dependent, depressed, weak, resentful, and all the more focused on her illness.

For these reasons J was ambivalent, but she decided to go ahead and apply to school. Given her history of learning difficulties, it was important for J to apply and be accepted to social-work school, but she then decided not to attend. In these years I was torn between interpreting the exhaustion J felt and her reluctance to pursue various careers requiring long-term commitments and "letting" her follow her instincts. The ever-present question is, "Is this resistance?" Should I view J's choice not to work or go to school full-time as a secondary gain from her illness enabled by her parents, or as a realistic, mature response to her health needs? If J had not become HIV-positive, she would have had many conflicts around career and self-sufficiency to resolve, but this was not the case. She was HIV-positive.

I no longer recall the way J found the unusual treatment modality she has pursued to this day. I think she first heard of it in California as a treatment for candida. Increasingly, J's intractable candida had become an ongoing reminder of illness and infection. When would the secretions end? When could she feel clean? As I recall, the first treatment took place in Toronto and precipitated a healing crisis that left her quite weak and disoriented on the subway as she made her way to the plane. The new treatment had even more restrictions than previous ones. There were homeopathic metal lollipops and transdermal patches that could be deactivated by radiation and electricity, so she couldn't go through the metal detectors at the airport. She needed weekly or biweekly treatment and at first it seemed she could only receive this treatment in

Canada. But J found people in New York who were conducting research on this technique and were willing to treat her. There were pills to take, a diet to follow, lollipops to suck for 15 minutes at a stretch, toxins to avoid, and injections to receive once or twice a week. The injections at times triggered memories of heroin, at other times they triggered healing crises. The frequent changes in treatment protocols, decided upon by unconventional means, stretched my credulity. With each new treatment modality, J would bring me literature and try to explain the rationale. She and Paul continued to get checked; Paul stayed HIV-negative and J's T cells continued to hover around 500. She had already had surgery for cervical dysplasia, and before starting this new treatment, she had been sick on and off for months. J's energy began to improve with this treatment.

Looking back on those years, it seems to me that there was an inexorable rhythm. Was it a pattern? I'm not sure. J's health would improve, would be in the background for a time, and we would address career and relationship issues. But often we had not much chance to make headway before health concerns intervened again. Was this resistance? Who could argue with it? There was no question what took precedence. Every sniffle, stomach problem, each increase in fatigue understandably caused alarm.

Later that year, J's T cells dropped close to 400. I was becoming alarmed and wondered if she shouldn't consider AZT. She had had several consultations with experts in the field before we began work and often had felt disrespected and poorly treated. J was psychologically and viscerally opposed to allopathic treatment and Western doctors. She and Paul had decided to take a trip to Spain. Was this crazy and self-destructive? How much should I interpret or try to dissuade her? At the time, AZT was widely in use, but some people argued that it was very toxic and only provided temporary relief, so there was good reason to avoid it. I raised my concerns, but J argued that she sensed my pessimism and alarm and this attitude wasn't good for her. She knew that I meant well, but she was concerned about the impact of my negativity. She and Paul left for Spain.

J came back with an extraordinary tale of psychic surgery in Ibiza, a ceremony that she didn't understand and that scared her considerably; but when she was tested upon her return, her T cells were up to 775, significantly higher than they had been for over a year.

The psychic surgery was performed at night by a Brazilian healer, surrounded by onlookers. J was very frightened as he threaded something through her throat, and she felt sick and weak the next day. This experience left us both with a respect for things we don't understand, that don't make rational sense. I still have my moments of doubt. For example, J recently told me that the homeopathic practitioners had asked a psychic to channel Frank, the discoverer of this treatment, to ask him why J wasn't improving more rapidly. "Frank" commented on how she had been neglecting her health and her diet and had to focus on eliminating parasites and fungus. He also was concerned about her stress about her disease and her sadness over her desire for children. It's true that J had been relaxing her stringent lifestyle, enjoying some alcohol, staying up late, in many ways pretending she wasn't positive. But channeling! Am I really sitting in the room, nodding in agreement with the advice that has been arrived at through channeling? What would my friends, colleagues, and former supervisors say?

I don't know what J will do if her health deteriorates. I have come to respect the complexity with which she evaluates treatment issues. Recently J's husband expressed his concern about her health, and with a renewed sense of urgency asked that she give him medical power of attorney. Consciously he fears that if J were in the hospital dying, her parents would wrest control over her treatment and make her take drugs. He wanted to be sure that he would have the authority to keep her medication-free. J said to me, "Gee—I don't know that I'll want to be medication-free. Certainly if I'm in pain I want morphine."

With each new claim that hits the papers, for example, the success of protease inhibitors, I have a renewed sense of anxiety that I'm not doing my job right, that it's crazy not to take these medications, and that I should be working through J's insistence on going the natural route. I do bring up reports that I read on new medications and ask her what she knows about them, what she thinks. She is always informed about these new allopathic treatments, but to date has had serious reservations and criticisms.

Paul's work increasingly took him to California, and in 1993 they moved. J and I continued to have periodic phone sessions and would see each other when she came to New York. The phone sessions were an unsatisfactory compromise but seemed the best we could do. J's life was relatively stable, her health was good, and she was working on a movie about being HIV-positive. As long as J had a creative project and was healthy, she was happy. In fact, one of the alternative healers she had gone to specifically counseled that she must stay involved in creative work or she would get sick.

Life and death continued. While working with J, a patient of mine died of an accidental overdose of heroin, right after leaving a detox program. Another patient's cancer returned, just after the five-year-clean anniversary. It came back with a vengeance. She died in November 1995. J's aunt was diagnosed with cancer and died, leaving small children, and then her grandmother died. Our mortality remains a steady backdrop to all we do. The only questions are when? how? what should we do while we're here?

In California, J made a movie. In it, she and a childhood friend frolic in the waves, dance, confront death. J is buried in a grave that is filled with leaves and vines. She rises and pulls an endless string from her mouth. This movie was harder work than J expected and was deeply satisfying. But what next? What story could follow the last one? As this question hovered, J's friend and partner in HIV, Beryl, got into a lot of trouble, and for the next several months J dedicated herself to helping her friend through this time. They became closer and, unlike the women that J had met in HIV groups before, they had a lot in common besides HIV, and, unlike J's other friends, they had HIV in common.

A somewhat reckless adventure ensued. The only warning I had of this came earlier in California, when J went to a doctor to have a wart removed and didn't tell him her HIV status. I questioned her, and the response was, "Well, he was taking universal precautions anyway; he asked if I was sick with anything. I knew what he meant, but I'm not sick now, so I said no." This was unusual for J, and we spoke of her desire just to forget about the HIV, to be normal, to not have to explain. I didn't anticipate the way this intense desire to be "normal" could play itself out until I got a distressed call for an appointment. J and Beryl had been spending a lot of time abroad lately, away from their husbands, and had become exceedingly close—buddies like in the old days. J arrived in my office looking great, tan and radiant, but she was also distressed and agitated.

"Beryl is having an affair. I can't believe it, it's so trite. Beryl doesn't want to hurt her husband but says it was incredible. . . . She was even able to paint again. I can't believe she's doing this . . . I kind of envy her."

Central to this affair was that her lover didn't know that Beryl was HIV-positive. At first, J didn't understand my reaction to her friend's behavior and insisted that Beryl had made sure they were safe. J insisted that the only thing that bothered her was the idea that Beryl could so easily jeopardize her marriage and seemed to be having so much fun. It reminded J of her own behavior in her teens and early 20s, and she wondered if she would ever have fun like that again. Gradually it became clear that in the affair Beryl acted as though she was back in time, pre-HIV, sexy, free, reckless, drinking, partying. Beryl rationalized her behavior, claiming that she consciously withheld something from the man in the affair so that she could keep something that was just between her and her husband.

I was quite distressed and judgmental about Beryl's behavior, and I worried that J was focusing on this as a way to warn me that she too was tempted in this direction. I could certainly appreciate J's envy and her desire to feel free once again. But given J's HIV status, thoughts of an affair seven years into a relationship were both "typical" and extraordinary. In this case, these fantasies expressed not only the typical desire of married people to once again experience the thrill of a new romance, but also expressed a most powerful desire to be out from under the weight of being HIV-positive. For now, J seemed content to live vicariously through Beryl, and she had been inspired by her friend's affair to write songs, not only of impossible, doomed love, but also deeply felt songs about life and death and her joy at moments of being alive.

J loved Paul, didn't want to hurt him, and was very upset by the lesson she was learning from Beryl. She saw how easy it could be to destroy a marriage—Beryl's was coming undone. She knew that her friend's affair grew out of some powerful dissatisfactions and gaps within her relationship, and she feared that the same thing could happen in her marriage if she and Paul didn't pay closer attention to some difficulties that they were having.

I was impressed with the way J worked on these anxieties with Paul. J and Paul moved back to New York and she got back into more intensive treatment. Paul realized that there were issues between them that had to get resolved and he began individual therapy.

Big problems remain: J continues to feel unsettled professionally and longs for more intensity in her marriage. The emotional and sexual frustrations that color J and Paul's relationship are not uncommon among the women I see in my practice, and J is more determined and inventive than many at seeking solutions. They don't have the option that many couples at this stage would choose—they can't have a biological child together yet. Beryl had gotten pregnant several years ago and her T cells had plummeted. J desperately wants a baby, and in her thoughts and dreams it is clear that this understandable next step would, at least for a time, reinvigorate her marriage. Were it not for the risk to J's health, she might be willing to accept the odds of her baby being sick, but the risk to her own health is too great. Paul doesn't want to talk about adoption, I think he feels burdened enough by his concerns about J's health.

When J speaks of babies—or of looking for a bigger apartment—there is a sense of future. Maybe in a couple of years there will be children. Some days we spend most of the session with that sense of infinite future; the next session we might be speaking of living wills. I follow J's lead in this; she's done more thinking about her own mortality than most people, and the sense of uncertainty is always there.

My work with J has made me reconsider and reevaluate some of my prior assumptions as a psychoanalyst. I became aware of the extent to which the collective denial of death permeates our field. Psychoanalysis, with its interest in psychosomatic diseases, gave weight to the belief that if we thought the right thoughts and dealt properly with our emotions we could avoid a great many diseases. Even cancer and heart disease were seen by some analysts as consequences of repressed anger, sexuality, or other intense affects. While the depression-stress-immunity links are real, so are germs, viruses, and genes. Psychoanalysis can help in many ways, but it does not make us immortal, does not make us omnipotent, does not give us an invisible shield against external and internal agents of destruction, nor does it free us from our individual limitations and heredity.

We don't need to posit a death instinct; we don't have to posit an instinct that we either work with or are conflicted about. We're going to die, no matter what. Even that oft-cited cliché—the only certainties are death and taxes—is a form of denial. We all know that we can cheat on taxes—does that mean we can cheat death? Since the 1930s in this country, death and dying have become more closeted—locked away in hospitals, hurried through basement corridors in body bags, easier to deny. AIDS forces us back to reality.

The denial of death within the practice of psychoanalysis is ironic, inasmuch as Freud, our founding father, lived with chronic pain and fear of death for the last 15 years of his life. Imagine for a moment that Freud were your patient in 1924. He is told he has cancer of the jaw and must have surgery. He continues smoking. As his analyst, do you interpret his self-destructiveness, do you suggest that he alter his expectations of life, that he reconsider his priorities? What is it like working with someone you expect might die during the course of treatment? In fact, Freud coped by cutting down on his social life so that he could continue seeing six patients a day. He found it so painful to speak that it was difficult to do much more than see his patients. He continued to think and write and teach, but he had his daughter Anna read his scientific papers.

Freud thought about dying and worried about his health. Often on his birthdays he would write to friends that he expected it to be his last year.

An interesting scenario: you are looking for an analyst in 1929. You consult with a friend who is in the field. She knows that you want to work with the great master, with Freud, but senses that you may need a long analysis, and she knows that he has cancer. She refers you instead to a younger man, Sandor Ferenczi. He dies in 1933 while you are still in treatment with him and in the midst of a deep regression.

My point is simply that no one knows when he or a significant other will die. We usually don't willingly choose to get deeply involved with someone who will soon die, but we never know. We think we're sensibly evaluating situations by some preconscious knowledge of probabilities—after all, it's the best we can do. During the time that I've worked with J, two other patients of mine and one analyst have died.

We never know. We try to manage our fears about mortality in both sensible and irrational ways, but we never know. Psychoanalytic treatment, like all our other endeavors, must survive the paradox; we make plans as though we can know our future, but each moment can be our last.

Working with J forced me to look at my prejudices and secret assumptions about what constitutes a rich and fulfilling life. For Freud, this was work and love—a reasonable bourgeois ideal. For many of us it still is, but increasingly for young people meaningful work is once again a questionable option. Meaningful work is a relatively recent and local goal. So, for that matter, is romantic love. And yet, as psychoanalysts we often act as though these are the only appropriate goals, the only ends that make our lives or our patients' lives worthwhile. Failure to achieve these goals often is seen as a personal and psychological (read *moral*) failure. I think that as analysts we must try to confront these preconceptions honestly—not reinforce them. Muriel Dimen and I led a workshop on just this topic years ago. What do we secretly believe is normal and healthy? What outcomes of treatment are seen as "cures" or successes? Many people, not only people with AIDS facing an early death, may find different avenues for self-fulfillment than those we or they traditionally expected. The values of personal integrity, love, and human attachment that Mark Blechner referred to at the 1996 White Institute HIV conference may find expression in many different forms. Or, as many Buddhist teachers point out, a close encounter with death can focus the mind on greater spiritual truths. For now, J and I continue, one day at a time, in the space between birth and death.

6 Psychotherapy of an AIDS Patient with Dementia

Karen Marisak

Psychotherapy and dementia seem unlikely companions. Can psychotherapy be of use to someone increasingly impaired by dementia? If so, what might that psychotherapy be like? What follows is a summary of my experience doing once-a-week psychotherapy for about one year with a 43-year-old man with AIDS. He was a former health-care professional who was probably very mildly demented at the onset of treatment, but who became increasingly more so over the course of our work. For me, his condition and our work raised many questions, concerns, and reactions, the discussion of which I hope will be useful to others in similar treatment situations.

I began seeing Darryl in psychotherapy in early March 1994. He had been referred specifically to me a few weeks earlier by the HIV Clinical Service of the William Alanson White Institute because he was seen as "someone who needs a lot of support." Darryl had been diagnosed with a condition called progressive multifocal leukoencephalopathy (or PML) in August of 1993. According to literature that Darryl brought me, PML is a progressive demyelinating disease of the central nervous system that is opportunistic in immunocompromised individuals (Chappell, 1992). It is caused by a reactivation of a common papovavirus, the JC virus. It probably occurs in 5 to 7 percent of people with AIDS. Clinical signs of PML include generalized or localized weakness of one side of the body or limbs (sometimes very severe), blurred vision or loss of vision (sometimes only on one side), lethargy, and cognitive impairments that may include language impairments, memory loss, confusion, disorientation, and loss of balance. Symptoms usually progress rapidly and mortality is likely within a year after diagnosis. Some studies indicate a four-month mean survival rate. About 10 percent of people with PML recover with or without treatment, but some very new treatments are offering more hope.

When Darryl was diagnosed with the PML (provisionally by an MRI to look at brain lesions, and definitively by brain biopsy), he seemed mildly organic: misplacing things, forgetting people's names, experiencing some confusion and time disorientation. But by the time I met him, he had been undergoing, for about six months, a somewhat experimental treatment regime that entailed a week-long stay in the hospital each month for chemotherapy with a drug combination called Ara-C. According to his doctors (an internist, a neurologist, and a psychiatrist), by the time of my meeting him he had improved greatly and was at most only very mildly demented, specifically seeming somewhat concrete in his thinking. But his doctors were concerned about his emotional response, one doctor citing his reactive anxiety, another his reactive depression, which seemed improved with Ritalin, and the third describing Darryl as "an odd person . . . chronically depressed and a loner," but more depressed since his diagnosis. He was expected to have only one or two more rounds of chemotherapy.

From our first phone contact, Darryl impressed as being fragile, needy, and likable. He was weepy and seemed very frightened, expressing fears of death and loneliness. Before our first session, he called me again to ask my opinion: his psychiatrist had suggested he bring Bob, his ex-lover, ongoing best friend, and principal source of support, to his first session. What did I think? I asked what his thoughts, feelings, preferences were in the matter, and why he thought Dr. L had made the suggestion. He decided to think it over and discuss it with Bob, but said he believed that he was certainly competent to come on his own. In the meantime, he gave me permission to call the psychiatrist, as well as his neurologist and internist. In fact, he did not bring Bob to that first session, but the question about this and my subsequent contacts with his three doctors set the stage for my having a much greater involvement with people in his life, including friends and caregivers, than I would typically have in a therapy relationship.

When I first met Darryl he was a slender, nicely dressed, neatly groomed man of average height. He had the light brown complexion of someone of mixed racial background, sharp, chiseled-looking features, thinning, graying hair, and a short beard. Darryl had two principal reasons for wanting therapy. First, he was experiencing overwhelming fears and sadness around his PML. The prospects of his illness were terrifying: dementia, wasting, loss of mind, loss of control of his body, imminent death, and a terrible death at that. Second, he was plagued by loneliness since the breakup of a 10-year relationship the previous year. He still loved Bob. Although they no longer were lovers or lived together, Bob seemed to be a devoted friend, deeply helpful to Darryl during his illness. But Darryl was lonely at night and longed for a lover to be there for him. Furthermore, since the PML, he had had to stop working and go on disability. Darryl had worked for a public agency as a health-care professional for 21 years, a job that had kept him active, out and involved with the people he helped. Finally, the winter of his diagnosis (1993–94) had been cold and stormy, so that he was often homebound with his illness. He had the help of home aides who were with him for two shifts a day and he was getting a daily meal delivered to him. Raised Catholic, but for years attending a very liberal, progressive Protestant church, he had in recent months become fervently religious, returning to his Catholic roots for comfort and security.

Darryl's History

Darryl's early life had been far from easy. His parents' problems resulted in Darryl's being placed in one foster home from about ages two to three, and then in a second foster home from ages four to 16, this time with his sister who was one year his junior. He described his mother as mentally ill, psychotic, and paranoid, and as being often hospitalized. He described his father as an alcoholic, intrusive, difficult, and a pervert. Darryl had caught his father peeking through a keyhole at Darryl's sister (then a teenager) undressing, and Darryl told me that his father molested him as a teen, but he would never tell me how. His parents, in their mid-60s, remained together and leaned on him with their troubles even after he was diagnosed with PML, but they never showed any interest in him or offered him any support.

In contrast, Darryl's foster mother is a loving figure, but she was elderly and limited by the time of his illness. His foster father, dead for some years, was a cruel, nasty man. He was divorced by the foster mother after Darryl and his sister were gone. Darryl and his sister returned to their parents' house when he was 16 or 17 because they were fighting with their foster parents.

Darryl's 42-year-old sister was divorced and had a 12-year-old daughter. The sister had ongoing money problems despite her employment in office management and computer work, so Darryl paid for his niece's psychotherapy even after he was on disability. Darryl also had a 25-year-old brother, born when Darryl was 18. The brother was doing well and was a graduate student in education. He was never sent to foster care, but was instead raised by the parents. He and Darryl were not close, and Darryl did not like to see him because he had dreadlocks. I believe this related to Darryl's uneasiness about his racial identity, and it also reveals some rigidity.

The topic of race was an important one for Darryl. His father was black and his mother was white, though with some possible racial mix in her background (one of her parents was European, the other Caribbean). He expressed a dislike of his background and an even greater dislike for being labeled as black. He was disdainful of Bob's new lover, who was black. (Bob is white.)

Darryl was married for about six years as a young man (ages 19 through 25). I know very little about his ex-wife, other than that she is white and that she grew obese after their divorce. They met at a train station—she had just run away from a foster home—and he essentially took her in (she was 17, he was 19). She quickly became pregnant, and they had two children in rapid succession, a girl and a boy, both now in their 20s. Darryl's wife left him when he was becoming more actively gay, going out every night to bars and bathhouses, unable to stop himself, despite the guilt. He explained that he was actively gay from the start of their relationship, but he had wanted to deny it to himself and hide it from her. He felt she was right to end the marriage. Darryl maintained a relationship with his children and told me he was glad he did. They have lived in Florida since their mother's remarriage to a man Darryl believes was a good stepfather to them. Darryl saw his kids several times a year, flying them up for visits with him. Much to his joy, he became a grandfather in September 1994 when his son's girlfriend had a baby boy.

After his divorce, Darryl had several relationships with men, including three significant relationships, before Bob, with men who have since died of AIDS. When in his early 30s, he met Bob through a hiking club, and they dated for four years before living together for two years. They then lived apart, but they were still romantically involved until Bob broke up with him about six months before the diagnosis of PML.

Darryl attended Catholic schools while growing up, and he expressed gratitude to them for giving him structure, stability, support, and values. During high school, he considered studying to become a priest. Instead, he went to college, got a master's degree and then did some postmaster's training in his field. He had both hospital and community jobs, and his employments were quite lengthy.

Darryl learned he was HIV-positive several years before coming down with PML. Up until PML, his health had been good, though he had had one bout of pneumonia and surgical correction of anal fissures the year before.

Course of Treatment and Questions Related to It

During Darryl's first few months of treatment, there were some ironic turns in his state of health. The first came right away. He came into his second session with "wonderful news!" He said he was cured of PML. He had had an MRI three days before, and almost all of his brain lesions were gone. "My prayers have been answered!" I later spoke to his neurologist, who confirmed Darryl's report. Darryl's mood was, not surprisingly, dramatically improved. There was still something of a slowness to the sessions. He was not very spontaneous, did not elaborate much, was not interested in deep explorations. He could be mildly surprised at my questions at times, as if I should already know the answers. Whether this was a result of residual dementia or something characterological was something I could not know. I also wondered about the intense, almost childlike religiosity, but I saw it as a tremendous source of comfort for him and not as something to be questioned by me.

These early sessions were practical, supportive, and exploratory. Darryl talked about his past lovers who had died, some friends currently suffering with AIDS, his childhood, his family, his kids, his relationships with his friends, especially with Bob. There was a certain vitality as he explored ways to get back his life. For example, he was going to the gym, had joined a group at GMHC, placed a personal ad in the hopes of finding a new lover, joined a Fire Island rental group for part of the summer, and made other weekend and vacation travel plans. He canceled his home-delivered meals because they restricted his freedom.

Darry was troubled by impotence and difficulty ejaculating, and this loss compounded his loneliness. He feared it would make it all the more difficult to form a new sexual relationship. The impotence also interacted with his religious guilt. He knew that the Catholic Church condemned homosexuality, and so he had to grapple with a sense of wrongness and sin regarding his sexual desires, now that he was again fervently Catholic. But he tried to be more accepting of his sexual wishes, believing God would accept him as human.

Though lonely and longing to be involved and loved, Darryl told me that he would not want to be in a relationship with Bob again, even though he still loved him. Bob is too sensitive to criticism. He takes on responsibility for everything and so gets too upset if Darryl complains to him. Perhaps in a more open-ended analytic therapy, this finding fault with Bob and the assertion that he, Darryl, would not want the relationship back, would be fruitful grounds for exploration of Darryl's interpersonal and defensive style. But here I saw it as part of Darryl's reconciling himself to his losses and gaining a bolstering sense of mastery and control over his situation, which might prove useful in his sustaining himself in the face of further inevitable losses.

Once, when Darryl was not sure what to talk about, he questioned the relevance of the therapy. (Incidentally, he had been in therapy twice before, years ago, first when he was married and then when he was recently divorced, but he would never tell me much about those experiences.) He told me what he wanted now was to talk and feel supported by me. Perhaps not yet willing to accept this as final, I tried to explore with him what was going on between us, but Darryl did not want this. Instead, he reassured me that he liked me and felt comfortable. I found myself pursuing him with questions that he would answer, but without elaboration. Often his voice was hard to hear. Yet he assured me he was feeling okay. He asked about me: Am I married? Do I have children? I answered the questions straightforwardly. Again I would wonder what was going on. Was I seeing characterological features, resistance, avoidance, withholding, depression, or organically based rigidity? And what was the best way to proceed? My compromise was to ask a little, and then to respect his wish not to go further with something he found unpleasant.

In later sessions, Darryl asked other similar, basic questions about me, such as what my religion was and if I practiced it. Again, I answered. This basic knowledge of me became important over time as he became more demented. He would recite the details of what he knew about me, somewhat repetitively, almost every time we met. ("You have a 14-year-old son named Christopher. You're Catholic, but you don't go to church.") It seemed like landmarking or structuring. It was a way of feeling related. More important, perhaps it was a way of proving himself and of feeling in control.

Though he had been feeling and assuming he was all better, during our third month of treatment (our 13th session), Darryl told me he was having some memory problems, though much less so than when he was first diagnosed with PML. Now he was forgetting his keys, his tokens, and people's names occasionally. He was keeping active, however, and preferred to talk about his recent visit with his son and daughter. He wondered what diagnosis I would give him and suggested "adjustment reaction with mixed emotions." I did not disagree.

For the first time, Darryl missed his next session. I called him and left a message on his machine. His return call confirmed an incorrect next-appointment time, so I then called him back. When he came for the next session, he explained his prior absence: He had tried to come for the session but had gotten lost. He found himself not knowing where he was, but he finally figured out how to get back home. He didn't know how it happened. He said, "I thought I was going crazy." At the insistence of Bob and another good friend, Mike, he was going for an MRI scheduled by his internist. In the meantime, his neurologist was being reassuring. Darryl's mood at this point was very positive. He was feeling enormously better, credited his therapy, and had many activities planned to which he was looking forward. His T-cell count had climbed from 84, when I first met him, to 124 in the prior month, and to 162 in the current month.

When he came to the next session he was traveling with his home aide, at Bob and Mike's insistence, because of recent forgetfulness. For the same reason, he was also in the middle of a neurological workup. His spirits were good, however, and he did not seem to give much importance to what was happening. I remember feeling grateful that he had his close friends, who were so actively involved, and that his doctors seemed to be right on top of the situation. I spoke with his internist later that day and with Bob later that week. Both wanted to tell me the same thing: Darryl probably now had AIDS dementia and not PML, and this was likely to mean a progressively downward course over the next few months, as Darryl lost more and more of his abilities, and needed more and more custodial care, until he would finally fall into a coma and die. So, here was the second twist: Although the PML was cured, the outcome for Darryl was likely to be the same. He had a new disease, without the specific brain changes of PML and without PML's known viral cause, but with a similarly devastating likely clinical course.

Darryl did proceed to change very gradually over the next few months, although he never reexperienced the devastating emotional crash that he had experienced when he was told he had PML. Instead, he maintained a fairly strong denial about what was going on, as he became less and less competent and more and more under other people's control and direction. He could see what was happening, talk about it and complain about it, and yet he could maintain the belief that nothing was wrong with him. To my knowledge, no one ever told him that he had AIDS dementia, and he didn't ask, at least initially. Some months into his deterioration he repeated to me his diagnosis question, and again he told me he thought he had an adjustment reaction with mixed emotions; again, I did not express disagreement. It seemed to me the denial allowed him some measure of peace.

For a while, Darryl remained active, but he gradually started dropping out of most activities and spending more time at home. He had trouble sustaining interest, would get bored, restless. He would be annoyed that he could not travel alone. He was slightly more irritable, less tolerant. His weight shot up 40 pounds as eating became his favorite activity. But he almost never missed his therapy appointment.

Let me review the chronology so you can see how quickly things went for Darryl and our relationship. We started therapy in March 1994, just as he was on the brink of being considered cured of his PML. There was a flurry of health and activity, but by June he was noticing some memory loss, and by July he was considered to have AIDS dementia. He soon had 24-hour home care and a very sedentary life. By October, Bob was considering nursing-home placement for Darryl, but was hoping to delay it if he could get more outside support. By December, they had applied to the Cardinal Cooke Home, a long-term health-care facility for AIDS patients who are too ill to be maintained in their own homes, but Darryl refused to go after he saw it. Yet by January 1995, Darryl was willing to consider going to Rivington House, a new facility that he thought of as a home for men with AIDS, rather than as a nursing home. During those weeks he had become more childlike and sloppy (shirt untucked, laces untied, even food in his beard). He would mispronounce sounds, saying his Rs like Ws. And he engaged in some mildly disgusting behaviors, like scratching his dandruff (which somehow got to me more when he had shingles) and belching. His gait was often shuffling or unsteady. His alertness varied: he could be lethargic, or agitated and restless, or calmly alert.

We had our last session on March 9, 1995. The following week, I was called by Bob and by Darryl's aide. Darryl had run away. Friends were searching everywhere, and my office was one place he might turn up. He did turn up in a hospital a few days later, with a fracture in his arm. After the hospital stay, he was transferred to Rivington House. Though the therapy was officially over, I continued to see Darryl about once a month over the next six months, visiting him at Rivington House. He would call or write to me when he wanted to urge me to visit. In

August of 1995 he was hospitalized with pneumonia, when his children and his little grandson were up for a visit. I saw him three times in the hospital, when his physical and mental deterioration were dramatic. Darryl died in late October of 1995. Bob called me that morning to tell me, and I was able to attend the wake.

When I later reviewed my session notes in preparation for writing about this case, I found myself being surprised to see how unimpaired Darryl was at the beginning of our work. Similarly, I was surprised by the lively, healthy man I saw in the pictures of Darryl that friends brought to the wake. Later impressions take over to some extent, perhaps especially when the acquaintanceship is short. It seems to me that it takes a certain effort to hold on to a sense of this other person in his totality. While he is who he is in the present, he is also who he was in the past. But on the other hand, being too aware of how someone was in the past pits one against a tremendously painful sense of loss, of deprivation, of disappointment, when one is with a person who has become so altered.

I frequently wondered if I was doing the right thing in the treatment. It was important to Darryl to be there. He almost never missed his appointment. He even came once when I was on vacation, running away from his aide who tried to convince him I was away, and arriving at my office alone at the appointed time (this was at a point when the nursing-home plans were in process). In sessions, he was often unsure of what to talk about and grew restless and wanted to leave. Yet he also wanted to stay through the session and was happy if he could get past the agitation and stay. I would help by giving some reassurance and structure. I think he saw me as a support, as a source of positive feeling, and probably the very regularity of our meetings was reassuring—maybe even a link with normality. (When I visited him at Rivington House, we would stroll around the unit and he would proudly introduce me to staff members as his former psychologist.) I remember thinking at times that the content of our sessions was getting increasingly out of touch with the reality of his life. For example, we would be talking about his dreams of travel or his hopes for a new lover, and not about the fact that he had started wearing a diaper. Or we might talk about just one aspect of reality. For example, he complained bitterly at times about his no longer having control over his money since Bob had taken over, and he even said dramatically, "Well, he might as well just kill me then!" But he did not overtly address the reason for not being able to control his money—the more profound loss, the loss of control of his judgment, his loss of competence. The sessions gave him an outlet for his anger over changing aspects of his life. In his life outside the sessions, he made the concessions and accommodations that he had to make.

Yet, at other times we were quite embedded in his day-to-day reality. We spoke about how to get along better with his aides who angered him by controlling him. (He would announce, "I never hit my aides," and this would begin our discussion.) Or he would talk with some pleasure and relief about the funeral plans he had made, but he was worried that Bob and Mike were not helping him make burial arrangements, and he felt this needed to be done soon.

At times he brought up major life-and-death or identity issues. He would announce them, obviously troubled by them, but then he was unable or unwilling to say any more about them. For example, he would make such statements as "I wish I weren't gay." "I wish I weren't half black and half white." "I never think of killing my cat." "I never think of killing myself."

Sometimes he would regret his choice of profession, saying he should have become a priest instead. Usually the most I could do with these statements was to express interest and concern, perhaps question why he thought these things were coming up, and sometimes offer something vaguely interpretive or reassuring, such as, "I guess what you are going through makes you question some basic things about yourself" or "It sounds like you might be feeling bad (or mad)." Darryl would then move away from the topic.

Should I have challenged Darryl's denial more? Should I have more actively intervened in his life (sharing more of my observations with his caregivers, becoming more involved in the decisions they made for him)? Was our work together even psychotherapy? These questions, I think, are in response to the feeling of impotence, even of uselessness, that I had at times in the face of the terrible events that were unfolding in the lives of Darryl and his closest friends. I think that stepping out of my role would probably not have made me any more useful, and that challenging him more would have upset him pointlessly. That he chose to continue seeing me for as long as he was able suggests that my response was one that worked for him. But it meant always a certain uneasiness on my part, working with a sense of suspended goals and precarious good feeling.

References

Chappell, M. (1992), *PML Project Inform Fact Sheet.* San Francisco Project Inform.

7 "Playing with Fire"

Transference–Countertransference Configurations in the Treatment of a Sexually Compulsive HIV-Positive Gay Man

Jean Petrucelli

My patient, D, came to therapy with more strikes against him than most people. His primary presenting symptom was sexual compulsivity, but he also had been sexually abused by several members of his family, was exposed to extreme violence, had experienced prejudice for being gay, Hispanic, and poor, had a history of substance abuse—and he was HIV-positive. Sexual compulsivity was the main arena in which the transference-countertransference configurations were played out, but I also want to highlight the importance of basic human qualities in our interaction. We focused on shame, dissociation, self-regulation, and character issues, while never losing sight of the shadow of HIV in his life. Our interactions were intense and direct. I thought about cleaning up some of the language, but then realized this would change the character of what happens in the room; so please pardon my French.

History

D is a well-groomed, attractive, 27-year-old light-skinned Hispanic man, with a short and slight but once athletic build. D's HIV-positive status was first diagnosed when he was 16. The youngest of six, he has four brothers from three to 11 years older, and one sister five years older. D is the only member of the family not born in Puerto Rico. D's father is an alcoholic and was physically abusive to all members of the family.

D was sexually abused on a daily basis by three of his brothers from the age of eight through age 16. The brothers would make D perform fellatio on them or have anal sex with D as the receptor. D's role was always to please the other. If D cried they would beat him, make fun of him, or not speak to him. D said he understood this to be a form of love and desperately sought attention from his older brothers. He was willing to pay any price. D would say to his brothers, "I love you"; they would reply, "Suck my dick."

D also described seeing his sister have sex with his brothers. They would touch and play with her vagina. D recalls seeing his sister with her clothes off masturbating with a cat. D felt unable to tell his mother about his sexual abuse, because there was a tacit understanding that if his mother found out and told his father, father would beat and blame mother. No one within D's family has ever spoken about the sexual abuse. Now D's brothers are all married with children. Two brothers have been in and out of jail (one on a murder charge) and one was an IV drug user. It is not known whether any of them are HIV-positive. D is closest to his sister, and they are the only siblings who maintain contact with each other.

D's grandparents felt distant and ancient to him, although he was somewhat closer to his maternal grandmother than the others. There is a history of intergenerational sexual abuse. D's maternal grandfather, an alcoholic, would pull out his penis and ask D to play with it. Sometimes D's mother would see this happen and would yell, "Put that inside!" but that was the extent of her intervention.

Until the age of five, D lived in a three-bedroom apartment in Harlem. The five boys shared one bedroom. D was often sick with flu symptoms and asthma and recalls frequently being rushed to the hospital with asthma attacks. After kindergarten, the family moved to a better neighborhood in a nearby borough. It was a household full of arguments and physical violence, as well as sexual abuse. D's earliest memory is of seeing his father beat up one of his brothers, smashing his face into a glass window. He recalls seeing blood and the whole family running around in a panic. D describes another occasion when his father beat his sister with the handle of a machete. D's physical frailty was adaptive in these circumstances. He was generally protected from his father's physical violence. Once, his father shoved him under a bed so he'd be out of the way of father's own violence.

D claims not to remember much else of those years and is not clear who took care of him. Mother was depressed and tried to commit suicide many times. During one of her hospital stays, father took all six children up on the roof and said, "We are all going to jump because your mother left." D remembers crying and saying good-bye to his siblings. D tried to be protective of his mother who was often crying in her rocking chair. Once D offered to get a hit man to kill his dad. D often tried in vain to comfort and reassure his mother, but he would wind up in his room, as he states, "crying or jerking off."

D revealed to his mother at 16 that he was gay and moved out the next day. He said, "I have something to tell you." She said, "You like boys." He said, "It's more than that . . . to make it easier on you, I'm going to leave." D felt that her knowing would put tremendous pressure on her because she, as well as he, would be blamed and beaten by father. D's father had ridiculed gay culture in a hostile manner.

D did well in school, receiving straight A's and awards for outstanding performance in high school. He was on the bowling team and was the senior class president. He proudly told me he was on the cover of his yearbook. It was during high school that D was diagnosed as being HIV-positive. He was 16 years old and had never heard of AIDS. During his second sexual relationship with a male outside of his sexual abuse history, D and his lover were tested for gonorrhea, which they both had. The clinic doctor suggested they take this HTLV-III test (which is what it was called then) because it was "out for gays." They both agreed.

D was told over the phone that he was HIV-positive and that this meant he had a fatal illness. D stood on a bridge in New York City and said to himself, "God push me . . . I need to get out of this . . . I was just told I was going to die." Why he came off the bridge is not clear to D, but he proceeded to buy some angel dust from his brother and ended up on the bridge again, this time high and hallucinating. It is still a mystery to D how and why he didn't jump. He remembers feeling very scared and thinking that if anything happened to him it would hurt his mother. He also felt that he was being punished for leaving the family, for being gay, and for being sexual.

D's mother died of stomach cancer two years before he began psychotherapy. D spent the year before her diagnosis taking her to emergency rooms, where she was repeatedly misdiagnosed. D's sister intervened and took their mother upstate. It was there she was correctly diagnosed, became ill, and died. D attempted to comfort his mother by saying, "Give me your disease and I'll die for you," and he often has feelings now of wanting to pass away to be with her. They became close during her last two years, cooking together and hanging out with his friends.

Prior to beginning psychotherapy, D's T-cell count was 207. He made a decision not to be tested again for a while. Two years later, in 1996, D's T-cell count was 156. He tried AZT and DDI and participated in several research studies. During that time he became very sick, had constant fatigue, lost 25 pounds, and had severe bouts of diarrhea. He now prefers a holistic approach, with herbs, vitamins, O2, and Reiki and Chi Kung exercises. He sees a chiropractor in addition to his treatment with me. D feels that his physical health has improved. Although he sometimes suffers from fatigue, D feels his most serious and troublesome symptom is the reoccurrence of genital herpes on his penis, around his anus, and on his upper thighs. The herpes, lasting about a week, is extremely painful. He treats it with topical Zovirax.

When D began treatment, he was living with a male roommate, with whom he often had sex, although he was not D's boyfriend. D has been in a three-year relationship with a man, whom I'll call L. The last time L tested for HIV was about a year ago, and he was negative. L is aware of D's HIV-positive status, and up until the past six months they often did not practice safe sex. Six months ago, D got his own apartment and L "unofficially" lives with him. D had felt hesitant to make that commitment. D often has difficulty enjoying sex with his boyfriend, and reports feeling "dirty."

TREATMENT

The Issue of Humanness

D's first comment to me was that he has a problem with commitment. He then gave me the history of his two previous treatments, both less than six months, and we outlined some of the major issues that he felt he wanted to work on. He appeared nervous and presented in a manner that flipped from cute and endearing to pensive, but grinning at the same time. I felt that I couldn't get a clear sense of him, but there was something about his style that intrigued me. He also seemed determined and greatly relieved to be in therapy.

Near the end of the first session, I asked if he had any thoughts, feelings, or reactions to what it felt like to be here speaking with me, and whether he felt we could work together. I had felt that it had gone well, that we had covered a lot of ground, and had even done a bit of analytically oriented work. Without skipping a beat, he told me he wanted to begin treatment with me based on my greeting, handshake, and warm smile (so much for all my training). I had met him in the waiting room, and I shook his hand as I would greet any new patient. He said he was relieved to be speaking with someone who treated him like a human being and he then proceeded to describe his previous treatment experiences. The first was at a clinic, with a gay male therapist who D felt was nonresponsive. D would leave the sessions feeling destroyed, not having been able to tell the therapist what he was feeling. The second treatment was with an older woman, also from an agency. When D described his sexual compulsiveness and acting-out behavior, she shook her finger at him and said, "You can't do that." I had two reactions. First, I was struck by the punitive nature of her remark. Second, I became self-conscious of my own Italian ethnic inclination to use my hands, and had a strong urge to sit on them.

D's desire to control my responses was clear. If I were too laid back or came on too strong or was moralistic, I would lose him, so finding the right or acceptable stance would be a large part of our work. Looking back on this first session, I wondered if I would consider his warnings as typical, stemming from his character, or as a more particular need for me to be cautious, knowing we would discuss his HIV status and behavior in this treatment.

Whereas a patient may be anxious about his therapist's being human or an automaton, I suspect this takes on another shade of meaning for a patient facing a life-threatening illness. How much is he seeking a basic humanness? How much does he need extra assurance that I will not make him more anxious by bringing up illness, death, and destructive behavior before he is ready? While it was compelling, I couldn't assume that his warning to me was just a transference manifestation of his wish to control the other. I had to consider his fear and his need to keep me at a distance concerning his health status as well. It made me wonder in what ways a therapist's clinical stance and the analysis of countertransference and transference are affected by the awareness that a patient faces a life-threatening illness.

After about a month of meeting once a week, and a particularly painful session regarding D's mother's death, he missed an appointment. He called and explained he had severe diarrhea and was afraid to go out. He then called to cancel the next appointment, leaving a message 15 minutes before his session which said, "Please give me a call. I'm having a hard time getting back to your office. I will be here during our session. If we could just talk for a few minutes it would be wonderful. Until then, I hope everything is well." I called him and offered to have a phone session, in which I suggested we meet twice a week. He said he had been wondering about the same thing and felt relieved.

It was at this time that I was first asked to present this case at the William Alanson White Institute's monthly HIV clinical case conference, which I have to admit influenced my intervention. I had readily accepted D's cancellation due to his medical condition, although it was only partially true, and I had not pushed as I might have with another patient. I then wondered why I had not raised earlier the possibility of meeting twice a week.

In retrospect, there was an interplay between an HIV issue and resistance in his cancellations and my agreeing to have a phone session. But it was not clear when D might use my flexibility in the service of his defenses. Was I feeling overwhelmed and uneasy about my ability to use myself fully with him, by maintaining a degree of detachment? Or was I reluctant to become involved in this process with him? I wondered if this was in response to my feelings about D having HIV and the eventual loss. Or was I responding to D's character issues and my own internal conflict regarding D's sexual acting out? In my thinking, I suspended my moral judgments about his sexual behavior in an attempt to form an alliance and also get through to him in an indirect way, but was I more bothered than I thought? I was hoping that he would come to recognize his sexual activity as a reenactment of his rage, hostility, and identification with the aggressor in the face of his history of past helplessness and his feelings regarding HIV.

Sexual Compulsivity and Aggression

The treatment of a sexually compulsive acting-out patient is particularly challenging under any circumstance. Sex is a way of relating for D, the core of his idea of intimacy. It is the common pathway and release for all his affect, be it anger, frustration, pleasure or pain. The situation becomes far more complicated, however, for an HIV-positive patient with whom a sexual encounter can also be deadly. This raises many issues from a countertransferential viewpoint.

D started telling me about his sexual acting out in a very contradictory context. After two and a half months, he proudly brought his 11-year-old niece to meet me. She sat in the waiting room during the session. He enthusiastically described how he was watching her, taking care of her, feeding her, and how this helped him take better care of himself. He then went on to provide more examples from his history, giving details of how he had been sexually abused by a 13-year-old neighbor, by friends, and by a high school teacher. In the next session, he reported he had been so stimulated by discussing his sexuality that he had to act out after the session. He left his niece in the car and ran into the park, on the pretense of urinating, knowing he was going to have sex. A guy walked up to him and said, "Hi, how are you doing, man?" while touching himself. Without another word they began masturbating each other. D then said to me, "But that wasn't all I did," as if baiting me to probe for more graphic details.

I was concerned about his endangering himself, others, and his niece, and I was wondering if the sessions were too stimulating. Our discussions might be intensifying his affect in a way that required immediate discharge through compulsive sexual behavior. So I asked if he had had strong sexual feelings after other sessions and if he had acted on them. He replied that, yes, he had had anonymous sex after several sessions and felt disgusted, embarrassed, and ashamed. I inquired as to what kind of sex and what role he played. He replied that it was oral sex, as a receptor or an inserter, and that he never used protection. Sometimes it was anal intercourse, and then he used protection 95 percent of the time.

In an attempt to address the self-destructive aspect first, I asked if he was concerned about getting an STD and lowering his own resistance. Given how hard he works at being health conscious with diet, exercise, and other holistic treatments, it was striking how unconcerned he was. Ironically, D had made a point of telling me that before coming to the session he had given a talk on safe sex at a community center. He even wore a T-shirt with RUBBER UP FOR SAFETY spelled out in big black letters.

We also explored his difficulty with feeling and expressing anger, both historically and presently, and how his aggression was being dissociated and channeled through these sexual acts. He explained that the only way he feels he could regulate these compulsive acts is to stay away from the park. I said, "It's not just compulsive sex, you could masturbate. It's about directing your rage and aggression."

I then said, "You are potentially infecting people with a fatal illness." He replied, "You are the first person to say that to me—the first person to talk directly about this sex stuff. My roommate just tells me, 'Hey man, you'll get through it.'" I told him that bridging the gap between these various aspects of self—the responsible, conscientious, and diligent side and the side that says "fuck it all"—would be the therapeutic work ahead. This session left us both with a multitude of feelings. Although I was angry at the fact that he was potentially infecting people, I also felt a warmth and compassion in response to his vulnerability. D has a boyish quality that leaves me experiencing him as a "lost boy," hoping I'll be his Wendy. There's another but smaller part of my experience that leaves me skeptical of his sincerity, given my evolving sense of his character.

D explained that part of what he was recognizing was that although he wanted to come to the sessions, "It was harder to come." He was having so many more feelings now and was thinking about them rather than just acting on them. (I felt that his words "harder to come" implied that "coming to me" is a sexual act, and that having and thinking about feelings is the beginning of entering therapy, rather than having therapy as another sexual acting out.) For example, he said he realized how the reoccurrences of the herpes helped him, because when he has an outbreak he doesn't want to go to the park. It felt good not to have that compulsive pull, and feelings were coming up that he knew he had to deal with, like not wanting to put someone else in danger. He told me how surprised he was to have an experience with a friend in which they just talked for three hours instead of having sex, and how wonderful and connected he felt. He said it was an experience of intimacy without desire and without feeling that the other required something more sexual from him. He found it a great relief not to have that pressure.

D described an experience of having sexual feelings on the subway. In response, he had started thinking of where he could go, but then he said to himself, "Chill," and he hit the subway floor, doing push-ups. He was excited telling me this, and said, "It felt great." We began to explore how he feels like there is a monster inside of him, how he typically doesn't allow himself to feel good, and how quickly he must rid himself of good feelings. D found it particularly hard to leave this session, and when he stood up he said, "I feel hot." I said, "Push-ups" and pointed to the floor. We laughed.

Push-ups became a metaphor, as well as a concrete tool, for regulating D's feelings. Soon after, he described how, while in the park on the way to a session, he found himself having to make a decision. He could go through the fields in search of sex and be 15 minutes late, or he could walk in the other direction, where a Rastafarian musician was playing, and be on time. He chose to hear the musician and found himself doing push-ups to the music. He felt proud of his choice. I felt hopeful that he was now thinking that he had choices.

Treating a sexually compulsive, HIV-positive incest survivor, who had an abusive, alcoholic father and a depressed mother raises more questions than answers. It is not always clear to me why I choose one direction rather than another to explore. First, when I think about D as an incest survivor, many questions come up. How conditioned is he to be overly compliant in the treatment? Is he identifying with the aggressor when he goes into the park? Is he being aggressive toward me by going to the park right after our sessions? Originally, I wondered whether he was acting suicidally or homicidally, and then I realized that this was an artificial dichotomy and that he may be doing both.

It is not wild to speculate that he is seeking punishment for a life of sexually taboo behavior. And in a broader context, does he unconsciously feel he brought the sexual abuse and the HIV upon himself? Inasmuch as his sexual behavior is an expression of a death wish, is this reinforced by his consciously known wish to be reunited with his dead mother? What kind of guilt and anger does he harbor toward her? Guilt, because he couldn't protect or save her; anger, because she never protected him.

D's sexually compulsive behavior continues, but he is experiencing more of an internal conflict. He reported, in a guilty way, having anonymous sex during the first couple of weeks back from the August break of 1994 (four months into the therapy). When I tried to understand how his behavior might have been related to what was occurring within the sessions or to my vacation, I wondered whether he felt a pressure from me to be compliant. He replied that he doesn't feel me as a pressure, but more like I'm a guide or support through these painful emotions, and that therapy has in some way required him to be more honest with himself. The following sexual encounter captures this struggle.

He went to Prospect Park before a session, thinking he was going to "fool around." Then he told himself that he needed to take 20 minutes to listen to the birds and do Chi Kung exercises. Fifteen minutes into the exercises he started feeling "Hurry up! I need to go into the park." Then he did saliva exercises three times, in which the swishing of saliva metaphorically cleanses one's body (he demonstrated this for me). By the second one, he could not swallow and felt that he had failed his own test by not completing the exercise. He walked into the park and started touching himself in front of other guys who were also touching themselves. One man walked up to him and took out his penis. D then took out his and began masturbating (parallel playing). The guy then picked up his shirt, zipped up his pants, and walked away. D said, "It was weird, I was already feeling unattractive. I thought it was my sneakers. But then I realized I had no intention of having physical contact with him. I didn't want to touch him, and this guy probably wanted to be sucked." It occurred to me later that I had missed a shift in D's acting-out behavior. D was satisfied enough only to masturbate in the presence of another man, rather than engage in some kind of physical mutuality.

As time has gone on, I have realized that even within my original formulation there are different subphases that can track the movement of D's sexual behavior from autoerotic to symbolization. These emerging shifts demonstrate how D's increasing awareness has facilitated the process of symbolization. An early sign of symbolization within the treatment occurred the week before the August break of 1995 (15 months into the treatment). D was struggling with wanting to stay connected to me without it being physical. He said, "You know, I had this thought, I probably touched Jean P. once when she shook my hand the first session. Yet there's something very personal and deep here without it being physical. But at times, I want to hug you and feel grateful at the same time." I replied, "You can feel hugged with words and feel connected to me without the physical piece. You know you can have a feeling without having to act on it." D replied, "Yes, and it means so much to me."

It's difficult to tell whether the next vignette represents a shift that had been occurring, or whether something occurred in the transference-countertransference that caused the shift. But it was clear that something important had happened when D demonstrated that he could not only have symbolic intimacy, but could also take on my role as the helping other. D had distributed flyers offering to do massage. Although he had worked on men before, he had never given a woman a full body massage. He told this woman on the phone to bring a two-piece bathing suit. She showed up at his apartment, not knowing a thing about him. D said he saw himself in her, that she was putting herself in a situation that potentially could be dangerous. D was aware that she would have entertained having sex, but he realized that just because *she* had feelings, *he* didn't have to have them. I commented that I felt she was looking at him as a professional and trusting him. D said he identified with the abused victim and was also able to keep his boundaries clear. He had this thought in the waiting room before the session: his objective is for "45 minutes" to provide the best massage he can do.

I told him the "massage" he was giving to me was about our relationship and the boundaries here. I felt that the message was, in part, a recognition that I can't "fix" him, but he can enjoy being here (for 45 minutes) and get something out of it—that I can't take the HIV away, but I can still want to help him. D said, "It's working on intimacy that is not just sex. I don't think I ever really separated that before." I replied, "You can be physical and intimate and still not be overtly sexual."

This early symbolization was tenuous and proved not to hold during the summer break of 1995. On the first session back from the break, D enacted a sex scene with me. He had decided he would go to the park to cruise and entered a public restroom. There was an older Russian man in the restroom, who began staring at D's penis, which was now erect. D decided to ignore him, left, and sat on a park bench, reading. The Russian man walked by him and said, "It get hard, it get big." D ignored him. The Russian man said, "How big?" D replied, "7$^{1}/_{2}$ inches" (at this point in the session, D looked up at me). The Russian man said, "Can I see it?" D said, "No." The Russian man said, "You want money?"

D laughed at him and went back to his book. The Russian man left and said he would be back.

Now I'm thinking, how would my analyst react? Great, now I have to picture his $7^1/2$-inch penis in my head. Well, I suppose this is exactly what he wants me to do. After all, I went on vacation and I might have forgotten him, so he has to penetrate my mind. So I think, I'll just hold it (the thought) and see where he goes with this. I maintain my analytic neutrality and just nod.

D continued his story, telling me he left the park bench, walked into a public restroom, entered a private stall, masturbated, and that it felt great. I had the thought that after D showed me his $7^1/2$-inch penis he took matters into his own hands, and my response encouraged that. I said, "You took control of giving yourself pleasure . . . great." D replied, "It's only in retelling the story, though, that I can take in feeling good and recognize this is a major step for me. I really see how you have been there emotionally for me, and I'm glad your vacation is over."

While I found myself supporting D's pride in having refrained from acting out with another, I was also aware of D's transferential need to please me and report good news. I found myself asking, "So what else is still going on that you don't want to tell me?" D smiled and told me there have been times when he has had compulsive sex and hasn't told me. Then he described another sexual dynamic that gets played out with his boyfriend and that led him to question what his own erections are about.

D feels that his anxiety comes out of his suppression of his sexual self that has been connected to illness and disease. When I asked, "When do you feel sexy?" we discovered that he doesn't know why he gets an erection and doesn't have a sense of what feelings are connected to having an erection—there is just a sense of urgency. He is aware of feeling intruded upon when he is with his boyfriend and D has an erection, even though they are there to have sex. D says he feels angry and that his boyfriend is interfering with his sex. I feel that on some level I am also the intruder to D, interfering with his sex. D says that as soon as L leaves, he "jerks off." This is his way of getting out stuff that he cannot say to L.

In the transference, I wonder about how our talking about sex and my intruding on his sex cause D to act out more. I want to emphasize that in the work with sexually compulsive HIV-positive patients, *how* we speak about sex is important. To speak about sex without being judgmental, overly curious, or voyeuristic, and at the same time be free enough to get a detailed inquiry, can require great delicacy. It has been helpful for me to join my patients through their own words, trying not to be seductive or voyeuristic. At the same time, I am aware of monitoring my own feelings to see if I am being seduced or stimulated.

Keeping this in mind, I approached the delicate subject of D's erections and his own confusion about what excites him. D says, "I feel like I have to do something with the erection." I asked him if he has ever thought of using fantasy instead of acting out. D maintained that when he sees flesh he feels an instant attraction. He looks at their penises first, then their faces. D consistently made the choice not to engage in compulsive sex. He described being at the gym where a man was touching his own penis in the shower. D got an erection, took a shower, and got dressed, realizing that he is an exhibitionist and a voyeur. D said he became aware and felt good when he knew the other person saw that he was aroused and was, in turn, aroused by watching D. D went on to explain in detail how he left the gym, walked to his subway, and found that "the sex thing is up." He said he had to hold on to his seat in order not to get off the train and cruise a restroom. He went straight home, however, and had "fabulous" sex with L. D said he realized that he can't live two lives. When he masturbates outside he feels dirty and different with L, and if he touches someone else he feels backed-off from L. He sighed and said, "Sex just happens" (like the saying, "Shit just happens"). I replied, "As opposed to experiencing desire, patience, and working toward something. It's again like things are being done to you—like the abuse."

I've come to understand D's use of sex as "the great connector." As such, I considered it an important step when D began using language and emotion as part of his attempt to connect—a greater move towards intimacy. Similarly, the vignette that captures his symbolic melding of intimacy to sex seems to capture some increase in his holding capacity. It seems reasonable to speculate that as he develops greater object constancy through the transference-countertransference enactments in our work together he will have yet more options. For instance, on the first session back from an August break, D told me how much he had missed coming here; so many emotions continually came up, and this was the place where he could deal with them. He said he felt confused and scared but tried to stay with all the feelings. My absence raised his fear of really feeling alone, and he retreated from friends.

D also recognized he was angry at me and then said, "This is the shit I hate about therapy. They either get all these emotions going and they leave, or they get all my emotions up and I'm left not knowing what to do with them." He continued, "But it's good to be here and see you and smell this office." The way in which he said "smell this office" struck me. I was fairly certain I hadn't overdosed on my Tres Jour that day, although I was aware that I might still be in a vacation mode. I wound up thinking about how nonverbal and basic his connection to me is.

Needless to say, D's difficulties do not exist in only one dimension, and so it will be necessary for shifts to occur in other areas where he has difficulties. Another area of concern has been D's difficulty in regulating aggression.

Sexual Compulsivity and Aggression Issues

D often reports his sexually compulsive acting-out behavior in ways that directly demonstrate his aggression within the therapy. In one session, D told me he wanted to cut back his therapy to once a week and, without a pause, said that he and L had unsafe sex. He allowed L to penetrate him without a rubber. D told me the conversation. He said to L, "You realize we did something unsafe." L answered, "Yes." I commented that they both colluded to do it, and I connected it to his wish to reduce his sessions. I inquired as to whether he felt that I had penetrated him in some unsafe way. It seemed obvious to me that his frustration with my inability to stop him from engaging in unsafe sex resulted in his saying, "Fuck you" to me. When he cannot address his angry feelings about me and the therapy directly, he will tell me about an outside event. D was unaware that this was an expression of his aggression.

As another example, D said, "I went to the park and did it for 45 seconds and then I pulled my penis out of his mouth and masturbated myself. Then I ran here to the session." I repeated "45 seconds—hum." He smiled and replied, "Yeah. I guess I need you to judge me without being punitive and wanted to know if you can accept me." I reinforced to him that I am not here to be his judge, but that I want to be able to welcome and speak to the part of him that is screaming to get my attention. He talked about his internalized, critical self that fills him with guilt, which feels unmanageable at times. We explored his feelings of guilt, anger, anxiety, frustration, and sadness in terms of the difficulties he encounters as he attempts to stay more conscious of these internal conflicts and states of unpleasantness. He said he was angry at times when he feels stripped of his ability to dissociate, or when he becomes aware of looking to me for solutions, or when he is faced with my limitations or humanness. He recently asked me, "Can you go through this with me? You too are human."

D then struggled with the limitations of our relationship and his anger that he cannot have more of me. He also told me he despised me for being there, listening to him, because when he feels like a bad person he feels undeserving of my acceptance.

When I ask D what it is he feels he is not getting from me in this treatment, he responds that I make him face things that are hard and challenging. It becomes overwhelming and too aggressive at times. Then he says, "But it's all my issue," to which I reply, "No, it's about us and the way in which we fall into this sadomasochistic pattern." D often appears to be able to take in and process what happens during our sessions. However, his apparent responsiveness can be misleading. We now explore D's difficulty with recognizing, or experiencing in the moment, feelings of being flooded, overwhelmed, or anxious. Without these regulating aspects visible to both of us, we have perpetuated a cycle where I inundate him and he adapts at a cost to himself.

In the transference, D often adapts to the perceived level of functioning. I understand his ability to adapt so readily as an expression of the way he survived growing up in a household of abuse. D remembered how scared he was of his father and recalled an incident when he had eaten some grapes from the fridge. Father lined up all the brothers except D and asked each one how many grapes they had had. Then the father hit everyone's hands with a belt.

Sexual Compulsivity and Self-Regulation Issues

One aspect of D's sexually compulsive behavior is his deficient capacity to self-regulate. Be it his impulses, mood, behavior, or relationships, he can swing wildly from one extreme to the other or can sometimes get stuck on one end of the spectrum. He struggles with feeling deficient in self-esteem and tension regulation. D often relies on external cues, like walking in the park or passing a subway restroom, to determine if he should have sex or not.

The sexually ritualized sequence of compulsive behavior may provide D a temporary sense of organization. His disturbing, vague, amorphous feelings that precede the compulsive sex act are then replaced by intensely felt affects that are easily attributable to a discrete event—the sex act. D feels guilty and hates a part of himself for doing it. Everything is explained by, or related to, the compulsive sex act. The sexual acting-out behavior becomes the central organizing event in his life and substitutes for a coherently organized set of goals and values.

Preceding the sexual act, D feels some sense of discomfort. It ranges among agitated restlessness, empty depression, unnerving excitement, or deflating disappointment. Part of how I utilize the concept of self-regulation with D involves an understanding of self-regulation as an interpersonally developed phenomenon. Alone, D struggles with his own capacity. The back and forth, holding, containing, and negotiating that goes on between us helps to enhance his underdeveloped function of regulation.

Shame

I have often wondered how my technique in treatment is affected by the knowledge that D is HIV-positive. I know I must be free to respond to D's behavior, remaining open and direct while not sounding punitive. Our talks and D's behavior were beginning to reflect that my maintaining a nonjudgmental stance, in part to prevent evoking his shame, was enabling D to make effective choices to take care of himself, which he claims he has never previously managed to do.

He said that when he thought about my saying, "Bring that dark side of you here," his first impulse was "I can't do that. It's too ugly." Then he thought, "This is how I need to figure out what this side of me is like, but it's painful to show you parts of me that I don't want to recognize." He said, "Sometimes I feel, what is it that you want? and what the hell am I doing here, if it's going to be painful? There's an underlying feeling of support here, and I can't figure it out. Your words come in my head, now, in the park, and I want to be here. But what am I giving you? I'm afraid even to ask you how you are doing or say 'Have a nice weekend.'"

We talked about D's difficulty having a relationship with boundaries and being in a position where the focus is on him. He was beginning to allow himself to experience more of an internal conflict, rather than to dissociate his feelings (like he did when he was abused). D was struggling and actively searching for the limits of our relationship, for example, struggling with the August breaks, calling when he needs to in between sessions, and not knowing what he could or could not ask for. He told me directly, "I don't feel entitled to ask for things . . . and I feel a lot of shame. The tapes that run in my head when I try to do anything positive are 'You can't do it . . . you won't be able to do it . . . no one else has done it in my family.'"

D's feelings of shame in regard to having HIV surfaced in a dramatic and poignant way. He had a Shiatsu massage with powerful suction cups that left bruises and marks all over his back. When he showed his boyfriend, the boyfriend freaked out and said, "You can't go to the beach like that," but D went and kept his shirt on. He explained to me that he was afraid people would think it was Kaposi's sarcoma (KS). Having those spots felt like he was screaming, "I have AIDS." So he waited until five o'clock, then took his shirt off and went swimming, feeling nervous the whole time. He feared that although the beach was fairly empty, if people saw him swimming they would leave the water or the lifeguard would ask him to leave. I commented that it seemed he was really feeling like he could contaminate others. He agreed and said that's why he waited so long to go swimming.

Sexually abused patients often feel terribly ashamed and afraid that the world will know and see them as damaged. An HIV-positive patient with KS is concretely visible as having a disease that many are ashamed of. This presents a technical distinction to consider: When do you interpret a patient's shame and fear and when do you recognize the reality of marks, or the projection of what will be in the future? You may interpret fantasy with the aim that when it encounters reality it will be found untrue. You interpret a reality, or a fantasy that overlaps with reality, with the aim of coming to terms with it as a reality. Typically, one would interpret a shame dynamic as how the world *could* look inside and see what's going on; it is no longer reasonable to talk this way with a patient in whom the world *will* be able to see what is going on.

Dissociation through Drug Abuse and Acting Out

In case things don't seem bad enough, D has a history of drug and alcohol abuse. He was able to quit all substances cold turkey, except for pot. In one session he looked particularly groggy, and I asked him if he was high. He explained that he smokes pot every day, throughout the day. He claims that pot helps block out thoughts about getting sick, that there are nights he's so scared he can't sleep. Sometimes he even goes fishing at the crack of dawn. We talked about D's waning energy level and how marijuana may, in fact, be making him feel less motivated and more depressed. I told him that I thought it was interesting that although he was able to give up all other drugs in the name of his health, he needed to keep this one. D, however, is able to reduce or stop his pot smoking for several months at a time.

I was struck with profound respect for how depressed D might become if he gave up all his acting out and directly reckoned with the meaning of both his history and his HIV infection. With that respect for his underlying depression, I became concerned that the quick shifts in D's behavior might be classified as a flight into health. I was reminded of that feeling of sitting on my hands. This is a highly impressionable man who is moving very fast in treatment. He has said directly, "I am very affected by words." He even got angry while listening to the weather report on the radio. The female broadcaster kept repeating, "There are clouds on the horizon." I wondered, given his HIV-positive status and depression, about how adaptive his defenses were and about my need to proceed with caution.

This was highlighted in a session when D reported his first dream and reenacted with me an emotionally dissociated experience of the previous week. For the first time, I felt he brought Strawberry Fields across Central Park West and into my office. In the dream, his mother was bedridden in the hospital, in pain and about to die. D was clearly emotionally connected to his feelings about the dream in telling it to me. With no verbal segue, he got a glazed look in his eyes and started telling me, more graphically than ever, a series of events that started in a Port Authority restroom.

D went into a stall with a door to urinate. A foul odor came up that shook and disgusted him. He thought, "Get me out of here" and wondered if that smell came from him. So he touched his penis and smelled his hands. D decided it wasn't him, so he zipped up, washed his hands, and left. He then walked by a restroom near the E train that he remembered as being locked for years, but it was now open. "Damn it," he said, upset that he now must go in. He interjected, "Meanwhile all this time I wasn't feeling sexual." D entered one of the stalls, this time leaving the door ajar. He started playing with himself, got an erection, did a quarter turn to the left so these two guys could see his erection. He pulled the door open a little bit more to show them. D heard a noise and closed the door. He left the stall and went to another part of the restroom where the same two guys were now playing with themselves. D took out his penis and masturbated, keeping his eyes intently focused on the other man's penis. He told me that he had an orgasm and at first felt obligated to stay until the other man finished, but then he changed his mind, said, "Fuck it," and left.

As he told me this story, he was staring intently at my face and I felt uncomfortable. At this moment, I was not feeling like "Wendy" with one of the lost boys. If not for this discomfort, I might have proceeded with a detailed inquiry about what exactly he was looking at. Instead I realized that D was reenacting with me the experience of anonymous connection in the park or restroom.

The talk of sex in the room with me was an attempt to dissociate from the more difficult sad feelings. He managed to talk to me about death and dying, but then he resorted to his familiar defense (sex as the common pathway for all affect). He was dissociated from his sadness, yet highly connected to me in an alternative enactment. This connection also had an aggressive aspect. I felt I was being forced to be a voyeur, as if I too was in the subway restroom.

As suddenly as it had come on, D's dissociated, glazed look left. His voice changed and he said, "I had thoughts this morning that I wanted to die." He then shared an obituary, written for himself in a workshop several months before. It said "D died today of non-AIDS related causes. Although he struggled with HIV for many years, he dedicated his life to understanding the parts of himself that were not part of the HIV illness." I replied that I understood this as his attempt to think of himself as a human person with HIV rather than as an HIV person.

Summary

Throughout the course of this work, I have thought about the benefits and pitfalls of thinking of HIV as an organizer of how I see D and how D experiences himself. HIV does seem to have organized D and given him a sense of direction that he may not otherwise have had. Death does that for all of us, and a more imminent death may do it more imminently.

When this treatment began, D was very much out of touch with his internal states and could only sometimes identify a feeling of discomfort. As time progressed he has become more able to identify experiences and emotions. He is also now aware of how he connects these feelings to his "once automatic sexually compulsive behavior." When he has been able to recognize the underlying tension he can "stand outside of himself" and see that he has choices of how to respond.

In the treatment, I now know that when D tells me his story in a suspenseful way, he has chosen not to have sex. D may have shifted the seductive quality of the compulsive behavior to his storytelling techniques, but I no longer sit at the edge of my seat waiting for the punch line—does he have unprotected sex or does he make the choice not to? When he sexually acts out, there is no story. He just says what he did in his opening statement or he doesn't tell me at all. When he has been successful in his ability to be aware, recognize, and make another choice, he weaves the story in an energetic, dramatic, and seductive way. I have come to enjoy this foreplay, and we share in the climax of knowing a small battle has been won.

To give some idea of *D*'s experience of our work together, I conclude with a recent dream. D dreamt that the plant on his bedroom windowsill was talking to him. He said, "The leaves of the plant open up like an angel, with arms and wings extended." He got out of his chair and walked over to the palm tree in my office and pointed, "See, it looked just like this." He sat down and continued, "The plant said, 'Come on, you can fly.'" D replied to the plant, "But . . . one of my wings is chopped off." The plant said, "Open the window."

D explained to me, "The stem of the plant was tall, erect, so strong, confident, and grounded, and I thought, I'm planted, I'm grounded, I'm accepting that I'm grounded already. I feel I can face major obstacles." D went on to say, "When I got the plant as a gift two years ago it was a top without any roots. I had it in water for six months to a year till it got all these roots. Then I replanted it in soil, and it's been growing like crazy these last four months. The plant was shaped as an angel . . . wanting to fly . . . wanting to break out . . . needing help. I am searching to become confident and sure of myself, to be able to give to others without it hurting me. But there was a major block . . . and the window was closed. Can I open it myself? I'm trying to take responsibility for what happened to me in my life."

D continued: "At age eight, I didn't start the abuse but I had a part in it. I'm starting to look at my role in it. I got something from it, be it touch, love, compassion, and my taking that in affects me now. You know, dreams are incredibly visceral. I feel warmth in my body. The plant was so real, it was like you and I speaking here. The plant was like the eagle of strength—self-sufficient. I see a lot of strength here—you, your chair, your furniture, the picture of the angel you have in your cabinet. You know, I think I am the plant also . . . but I see the importance about getting help and nurturing it. Since that dream, I wake up feeling energized, feeling good. I feel like I'm doing my part, and I haven't done that in a long time. I look at the clouds and the sun peeks through. I was thinking, the dream is life that I'm starting to realize . . . I don't want to leave."

8 Managing Chronic Loss and Grief

Contrapuntal Needs of an AIDS Patient and His Therapist

Richard B. Gartner

Typically, an AIDS patient, particularly if he is gay, must prepare for his own death while dealing with chronic bereavement in his personal support system. As I write, in the late 1990s, most HIV-infected gay men—indeed most gay men, particularly those mature in years—have had multiple losses to the disease. Integrating these is quite a different matter from integrating the loss when a single loved one dies, or even when there are multiple discrete deaths in an individual's network. Coping with chronic loss and grief is tremendously difficult for anyone; for someone suffering from AIDS, such chronic mourning is potentially life-threatening.

One man I saw for a consultation shortly before he died was a long-term survivor, having lived 12 years with HIV, five of them with full-blown AIDS. It was wonderful in many ways that he had survived so well, but he told me with immense sadness that the only person currently in his life whom he had known for more than two years was his mother. Thus, he faced his death having a shared history with virtually no one but her. In addition, the loss of his entire personal network to the disease drastically affected his own ability to cope with his illness. It was an emotional drain on him, and it also forced him to realize there would be few people he could rely on in the final stages of his life.

As I considered what this man told me about his losses, I was shaken. How would *I* fare if there were no one in my life who had known me prior to two years ago? How would any of us fare under such traumatic conditions? And how can any of us bear to hear about such losses from people we grow to care about without becoming detached in our empathic stance?

By definition, the therapist working with AIDS patients also directly faces chronic loss; his or her job is to treat people with a drastically foreshortened life expectancy. Like the individual whose social network includes multiple losses to AIDS, the therapist with a large AIDS practice has to integrate, not just an occasional discrete loss, but an ongoing experience in which death can be expected recurrently in his or her professional life. For any therapist empathically attuned to his or her patients, such recurring losses exact a heavy psychic toll.

Thus the therapeutic work between an AIDS patient and a therapist experienced with this population is apt to have an unspoken counterpoint in which each has a need to deal with feelings of chronic loss and grief. Each may worry that the relationship will suffer because of his or her own problems in managing these feelings. The patient needs to work through the chronic mourning process, but may wonder whether it is possible to survive such grief work. Additionally, he or she may not be sure whether the therapist is up to the task of listening to it. The therapist needs to create a working relationship with the patient, but may have countertransferential problems about loss. Such problems, based on experiences in his or her own life or on those with other patients, past and present, may interfere with the ability to form an attachment to a patient who is likely to die while in treatment.

Managing the mutual concerns of this unspoken counterpoint to the therapeutic work is an essential task in such a treatment.

My work with Paul, a gay man living with AIDS who had suffered multiple losses to AIDS and other diseases and life events, prompted me to consider this issue during the 13 months I treated him in once-weekly psychotherapy before he died. The work with me helped him to reconsider his own life, much as any dying patient might do in therapy. But I saw that it also allowed him to ventilate his feelings of helplessness, grief, and rage about his chronic bereavements in such a way that he was able to elevate the quality of his life considerably in his final year—a year in which he continued to suffer nearly weekly losses to AIDS within his social network. Indeed, I believe that our work may well have bolstered his body's ability to handle the disease. This is supported by the fact that he was hospitalized for pneumonia three times in the eight months prior to the beginning of psychotherapy, but during our work he was in the hospital only once (for tests) prior to his final illness.

Loss echoed throughout our work and informed the intensity of our relationship. On his side, Paul was monitoring my ability to listen to the extent of his bereavement. On my side, hearing about Paul's losses, coupled with my knowledge that he, too, was likely to die, constantly affected how I listened to him. We worked in the context of our contrapuntal emotions evoked by loss.

Paul's Background

Paul was a 53-year-old gay man, white, and with a college education. The only child of comfortably well-off and conservative parents, Paul was raised in America's heartland, but had lived in New York City since his 20s. His parents died within nine months of one another in the late 1980s, one from cancer and the other in a car crash. Paul maintained little contact with his extended family on either side, and had inherited little from his parents, as they had suffered financial reversals in the years prior to their deaths.

Paul's Losses

Paul had had three major love relationships in his life; I will call them, in chronological order, Andrew, Bill, and Carlo. Paul and his first lover, Andrew, were together for 10 years. Andrew remained Paul's closest friend, and although not entirely in good health himself, Andrew had tested negative for HIV. Andrew and his current lover had promised to care for Paul in the final stages of his illness; this fact set Paul apart from the many AIDS patients who have no such assurances from longstanding friends or relations.

Paul's second lover, Bill, died of AIDS in 1984, after he and Paul had been together for seven years. Bill had been famous in several design fields, and together, Bill and Paul had led a high-profile and glamorous life. They had purchased a home that Bill decorated expensively, designing numerous articles expressly for Paul. Two close friends of Bill and Paul's were diagnosed with AIDS at about the same time Bill was, and both died within two weeks of Bill's death. These three were the first people in Paul's personal network to suffer from AIDS and to die of it. Their deaths marked a complete change in Paul's life trajectory.

This change intensified when both of Paul's parents died in the years following Bill's death. A man for whom interpersonal connections were very important, Paul once remarked that he had done far better in his relationships than in any other aspect of his life. But his personal network narrowed dramatically after Bill's death. He had been close to Bill's extended family, and he continued to relate warmly to them following Bill's death; but they lived in another country, so at the time treatment began, these relationships could only continue by phone, with visits every year or two. In addition, the many friends Paul shared with Bill faded from Paul's life after Bill died, remaining on pleasant but distant terms. Thus, in a short period of time, Paul's extended social and familial network became drastically smaller.

Paul did not get tested for HIV himself after Bill got sick. Like many gay men in the mid to late 1980s, he felt that finding he was positive for HIV would add to his depression without offering any treatment possibilities, since none were yet available. Nevertheless, he assumed he was indeed HIV-positive.

Two years after Bill died, Paul started a relationship with Carlo, his third lover. Carlo was a professional with a successful career. He had a large and warm extended family whose members seemed to accept Carlo's homosexuality and to welcome Paul into their midst. The life Paul led with Carlo was very satisfying to him, though it was quieter and more domestic than the glamorous life he had led with Bill. After three years, Carlo was diagnosed with AIDS, and he died two years later. Carlo's family quarrelled with Paul about Carlo's estate, and they asked him to leave Carlo's house, in which the two had lived together. Luckily, Paul had never given up the home he had shared with Bill, and so he was able to move back there. The nature of the quarrel with Carlo's family was never clear to me, but it seemed to have overtones of homophobia, as well as an unspoken belief that Paul had transmitted HIV to Carlo. In any case, Paul was devastated by the further loss of this familial network.

Professionally, Paul had "almost made it very big" in a highly competitive commercial field where youth is much prized. He had won awards, been highly paid, and had switched jobs often in the 1970s and 1980s, but he had never been successful in management positions. By the late 1980s, he had lost some jobs and had begun to make lateral job shifts, sometimes for lower pay. He was fired from his job about a month after Carlo's death and had not found a new one when he himself was diagnosed with AIDS four months later. He was therefore ineligible for disability at levels he would have received had he been working at the time of his diagnosis.

Within six months of his diagnosis, Paul decided not to seek further work. He considered himself retired and applied for support to various government programs, in addition to living off the capital from the estates of both Bill and Carlo. At this point, Paul became active in AIDS organizations like the Gay Men's Health Crisis (GMHC) and built up a personal network of gay men with AIDS. He was active socially during this period, a time when his physical health was relatively good.

Two years after Paul was first diagnosed, there was a major electrical fire in the home he had shared with Bill. This was especially traumatic because of the destruction of artifacts from Bill's life and most of the furniture and other articles Bill had designed for Paul. The home was ruined, and Paul had to live in a furnished sublet for eight months while the house was made liveable. Those of his possessions that were not completely burned were packed up and put in storage, many of them severely smoke-damaged. Paul was not in psychological shape to decide what could be salvaged.

As Psychotherapy Began

Shortly after Paul moved back home, he applied for psychotherapy at the HIV Clinical Service of the William Alanson White Institute. When asked why he wanted to be in therapy, Paul wrote: "My T cells have dropped to 61 and I'm having good days and bad days. I've lost many good friends. I need someone professional to deal with my growing awareness of my mortality and my concerns about my ability to deal with serious illness, discomfort, nausea, et cetera. Up until now it's been a piece of cake."

Paul had had several positive previous experiences with individual and group therapy. He had stopped these treatments, however, when his financial situation worsened and therapists were not willing to lower fees enough for him to continue. This had happened in the late 1980s, when he was in crisis following the death of Bill, and again after Carlo's diagnosis with AIDS.

Paul retained some bitterness toward these previous therapists, but he also expressed feelings of deep loss about the endings of his therapies. When I began to work with him, this was the first issue we addressed. He was eager to be in therapy, but he worried that there would be a repetition of the earlier abrupt endings because of money. His suspicions were raised when, because he had good insurance coverage, I set his fee higher than the minimal fee he had expected to pay. This caused an immediate minicrisis in the treatment: Was I going to take advantage of him? Was he going to get dependent on me, only to have me dump him if he couldn't pay later on? Did I care about him?

As we talked about his concerns, I began to get a measure of the man. I saw how he pressed me for answers without alienating me or minimizing his own emotional needs. His manner was direct and firm, but understated and not overtly challenging. Although Paul paid an emotional cost for dealing with the world this way, I also want to emphasize how he used himself positively to deal with his disease.

In particular, I was seeing in miniature how Paul had learned to mesh with the medical establishment and social agencies. For example, he had set up his medical care and insurance coverage with advice from AIDS organizations. He worked with a highly regarded internist specializing in AIDS care, but he was also eligible for treatment at the Veterans Administration, so he went there to get free medications, treatments, and tests. His routine was generally to see his own doctor first, then go to the V.A. and tell them what he'd been prescribed. When some V.A. doctors balked at being rubber stamps for the treatment prescribed by his private doctor, Paul developed skills to smooth their ruffled feathers and work the system to his advantage.

Had I been treating Paul in another context, and had he not been suffering from AIDS, I might have looked at these behaviors as representing some sociopathic trends in his personality, and perhaps in some measure they did. But as I got to know him, I saw his ability to confront and manipulate social systems as a strength, a kind of adaptive psychopathy that was in fact a healthy way of getting what he needed for survival in a difficult world. I therefore generally supported such behaviors and did not bring up negative interpretations of them.

Once we had discussed at length the frame of the treatment, including cost, we began to talk about Paul's life situation, mood, and state of mind. He had moved back into his apartment, which was now sparsely and simply furnished. Feeling overwhelmed by the task, Paul had not been able to get his smoke-damaged furniture out of storage to assess what could be repaired and decide how to dispose of the rest.

On the other hand, Paul was a part-owner of a summer house. While he could not afford his carrying charges, he was able to rent out his share in such a way that he could go there several times a summer and thus maintain relationships with people from that part of his life.

This summer home was very important to Paul as a means of

symbolically maintaining his former lifestyle. Similarly, he continued to garage a classic sports car for which he had little use; it did not function, and he did not think he could afford to repair it. He also continued to register for the New York City Marathon, in which he had run for many years. The last time he had competed in it he walked the whole way, which was simultaneously a moral victory for him and a sign of his mortality. Each year he sent in his registration again, knowing he could no longer run the marathon, or even walk it, but going through the registration process as a means of consciously maintaining a fiction that his life had not changed.

How Paul Used His Psychotherapy

Paul needed a place to mourn. He felt that at GMHC, where he now spent most of his time, there was a clear limit to how much people would tolerate talking about death. He had become careful about what he said, and to whom, about his friends all dying, because he was afraid of alienating people who had even more difficulty with loss than he, and thus further reducing his interpersonal network.

Paul took to the therapy with enthusiasm; it was the only place where he could talk about his many griefs, worries, and terrors. Therapy became the one safe haven where he could mourn, cry, and be fearful. Yet it was important to manage this in such a way that it was not the sole focus of our work—so that he would not be completely overwhelmed and could manage to keep some positive perspective on his life. There were many instances of this double process.

Paul had been part of a large network of friends at GMHC. He had been involved in many activities and attended theater and opera with these men. But when he began therapy, this close group of friends at GMHC was dwindling fast, as the men advanced into later stages of their illnesses and died. His two closest friends there were seriously ill, and over the course of Paul's treatment, both died difficult, lingering deaths.

This was a recurrent theme of the therapy, as Paul dealt with illnesses and deaths, month in and month out. He prided himself on his loyalty to friends and was often the only one in his personal network to visit men in hospitals or nursing homes. He spent hours on subways and buses to make these visits, sometimes finding that his friends were semicomatose or demented when he arrived. He voiced his agony about these visits in our sessions, and we talked through his feelings and fears. The nurturing he did on these trips was crucial to him because of both character issues and his escalating worries that no one would be there to see him through his own final illnesses.

This last issue was highlighted one day when Paul discovered that a man had died who, until a few months earlier, had run an important service in which Paul had participated at GMHC. A year before the man's death, this service had been active and vital. A large number of men, most of whom knew and liked the leader, had participated in it. But when Paul went into the crowded dining room at mealtime to tell people this popular man had died, he saw to his dismay that there was not a single person left there who had known the man. Paul was horrified to realize that he himself had survived most of the people who had cared about him, and he bleakly wondered whether anyone would remember him when he died.

When he was able at last to grieve openly in my presence, Paul's mood lifted, shortly after treatment began. The sessions were not, however, filled only with sadness; Paul was interested in the world, including the world beyond people with AIDS. He began to notice more psychological energy and even, at times, physical vigor. We then talked about the many practical problems of his life, and I helped him structure ways to prioritize and deal with them.

After a few months of treatment, he had his belongings brought out of storage, and he lived surrounded by boxes and smoke-damaged furniture for several months as he slowly sorted through it. He got rid of much of it, repaired some pieces, decided to live with or hide the defects of others, and sold the rest. These decisions became the meat of our sessions, as he told me the personal, sentimental, artistic, and aesthetic history of many of the pieces; I listened and helped him sort out what he could give up. For example, he had to come to terms with the fact that the furniture designed for him by Bill was no longer usable, with the exception of one chair that he could re-cover inexpensively. He gave up the unusable furniture after mourning once again the loss of Bill. This time the grieving took place in the context of having a relationship with me, and he seemed better able to move beyond it.

Giving up Bill's furniture ultimately had a very positive effect on Paul, as he recalled that his taste had always been simpler and less "drop-dead elegant" than Bill's. As we talked about how to put his apartment together again, it became much less a shrine to his relationship with Bill and more attuned to Paul's own current needs. For example, after we discussed his needs, he decided to put together a computer-oriented room that reflected his own areas of interest and expertise, and where he happily spent hours surfing the Internet and working on various projects.

Similarly, after we talked about it in a structured and pragmatic way, he had his car looked at by a mechanic and fixed; he decided not to sell it, despite the impracticality of keeping it and the rarity of his using it. He made plans about leaving it to a godchild who had once admired it, and he made other arrangements to dispose of his belongings after his death. As far as I could see, this was done, not out of depression, but as a way of reasserting some mastery in his life.

After 10 months of therapy, Paul was in relatively good health for a man with a confirmed diagnosis of AIDS. He had a chronic lung condition and cough, which had been revealed to be bacterial or fungal and amenable to treatment, though with limited success. There was no wasting; there had been no diagnosed opportunistic infections; and he had only had some relatively minor skin diseases. He did have occasional bowel accidents; he suffered great shame and feelings of humiliation about this, and wore special underwear to avoid having an obvious accident in public. Again, after he hesitantly voiced these feelings to me and we started to work them through, a pragmatic approach from me helped him begin to come to terms with this loss of function.

We also talked about how to marshal his waning strength. Paul reported that if he rested enough he could get done most of the things he wanted to. As soon as he lost any sleep, however, he got into trouble physically. For example, after spending all of Thanksgiving with Andrew's family and getting home at 10 P.M., he needed to sleep most of the remaining four-day weekend.

Three months before his own death, three of Paul's friends, including one of his closest buddies from GMHC, died over a single weekend. Paul counted up and realized that of the 20 or so men he had felt close to a year before, all were now dead except two, both of whom now had very serious medical problems. He was the only one in relatively good health.

Paul resisted making new friends at GMHC because many people there now were IV drug users for whom he felt little affinity, and also because he was afraid people would pull back from him when they found out how long he had been ill. Eventually, though, he began to connect to some newer members there, until he was hospitalized suddenly for an infection and began to deteriorate rapidly. I spoke to him several times on the phone and realized his contact with reality was quickly diminishing. Ten days after he was hospitalized, I received a call from Andrew telling me Paul had died.

The Therapeutic Relationship

Over the period we worked together, Paul became an enthusiastic supporter of psychotherapy for himself and others with AIDS. He felt, and

I agreed, that the therapy extended his life, and certainly raised its quality. He idealized me and the White Institute more, perhaps, than we deserved. When I asked him what was valuable about the work I did with him, he answered that I provided a place where he could say things he felt were unsayable anywhere else; that after we spoke, his life no longer seemed to be the chaotic maelstrom he usually experienced; and that I helped him see the shape as well as the value of his life history.

Yet I also felt he kept me at arm's length. For example, he always called me "Doctor" without using my last name. Likewise, he was startled and surprised by anything I did for him that he considered beyond my job, such as phone him in the hospital. Paul expressed virtually no curiosity about me personally, and when we explored this it became clear to me that he could not bring himself to ask questions that might make him see me as being vulnerable to HIV myself. Instead, he wanted to see me as healthy and without problems, particularly health problems that might lead to my being unable to work with him. This was even more pronounced after he heard a rumor that his internist was HIV-positive. For example, he did not want to know about my sexual orientation, although he did test me to make sure that I did not express heterosexist or homophobic ideas.

On my side, I was originally concerned that he might be envious of my presumed good health. I came to realize that this represented my own relief and guilt for being healthy in the face of a man dying in his prime. Later in the treatment, I admired Paul, perhaps excessively, for his ability to make his way through his emotional jungle without losing his own humanity, compassion, or sense of humor.

Managing Chronic Loss in the Transference and Countertransference

Injurious effects on the therapist who works with traumatized patients have been noted throughout the trauma literature, particularly the literature about working with sexual abuse. This has been referred to as "contact victimization" (Courtois, 1988), "traumatic countertransference" (Herman, 1992), and "vicarious traumatization" (McCann and Pearlman, 1990). Pearlman and Saakvitne (1995) call vicarious traumatization "a process through which the therapist's inner experience is negatively transformed through empathic engagement with clients' trauma material" (p. 279). They describe in some detail the theoretical underpinnings of the phenomenon, as well as its interaction with transference and countertransference and ways for the therapist to care for him- or herself in such circumstances.

Paul came to treatment in a deep depression. The multiple losses in his current life reverberated with his previous losses, so that an oscillating emotional reaction of grief was constantly with him. In addition, he had what struck me as a reality-based fear that the few people remaining in his social network would not be able to bear hearing the details of his feelings of desolation about his chronic losses. He needed and used the therapy as a safe place to ventilate these feelings and to come to some peace about his extraordinary life circumstances.

Like anyone else, I too came to the treatment with a personal history involving losses in my own life. In my case there had been a series of sudden deaths in my family that immediately preceded or followed happy family milestone events: weddings, bar mitzvahs, graduations, and births. A defining moment of my childhood was the postponement of my own bar mitzvah because of the tragic death of a young cousin in a car accident two days before the scheduled date.

Several of these losses were devastating to me at the time. My characteristic reaction had been to alternate between a dissociative sense that I was fine and hardly affected by such things and an anxious, hovering overattention to people's health and well-being. In recent years, I felt that I had generally worked through these reactions and that they rarely interfered in my work with patients. Nevertheless, I tended in my personal life to be wary when things seemed to be going exceptionally well, and I found myself worrying as milestone events approached and breathing a sigh of relief if everyone remained healthy afterwards.

Hearing about Paul's many losses stirred up these old griefs of mine, so that, as with Paul and *his* griefs, they reverberated in my experience as I listened to him. To imagine bearing such losses on a weekly basis was almost impossible for me, and when I had flashes of deep empathy for his situation I was shaken and stunned.

In addition, while I welcomed hearing about Paul's relative good health, echoes of my own history came up at times, and I found myself wondering if this good news was a signal that death was imminent. Would the usual boom soon fall on him, and hence on us? I rarely spoke to colleagues in the HIV Clinical Service about him or how well he was doing, and in retrospect I realize this was partly out of an unarticulated and irrational fear that doing so might invite a sudden worsening of his condition. Similarly, when I was invited to present my work with Paul to the monthly case conference of the HIV Clinical Service, I noted an anxious feeling inside that I might be inviting the evil eye on Paul by talking in positive terms about his treatment. (Indeed, Paul was hospitalized and died about three months later.)

I don't believe my countertransferential reactions were either extraordinary or damaging to the treatment. What was unusual was my heightened awareness of them. I don't know how much they affected my relationship with Paul. I do think he frequently surveyed my ability to listen to his losses, just as I surveyed whether he could express his feelings about them without falling apart. I also tracked my ability to listen to him, and had many internal dialogues about my own reactions to loss. From his commentary in sessions, it was clear that Paul had similar internal dialogues about himself.

Conclusion

None of us, neither patient nor therapist, is immune to the effects of loss, and certainly not to the traumatic effects of chronic loss. We may grieve openly or silently. We may work through our anger or sense of abandonment, or we may act it out in some way, or we may dissociate it so it goes underground, affecting us unconsciously with physical or psychological symptoms.

Paul and I became a dyad in which his experience elicited from each of us a reactivation of previous partly or mostly worked-through grief reactions. In the culture of our relationship, each of us continually monitored the other's ability to deal with the traumatic material Paul brought in, though this was not something we ever discussed explicitly. It was clear to both of us that our goal was for Paul to express feelings of grief and mourning in such a way that he (and I) could manage and live with them, rather than succumb to them. By acknowledging this separately and, to a lesser extent, mutually, we were able to do the mourning work Paul needed while not allowing it to be the sole focus of his treatment. Most important, we managed all the while to maintain a mutual and essential interconnectedness.

References

Courtois, C. (1988), *Healing the Incest Wound.* New York: Norton.

Herman, J. L. (1992), *Trauma and Recovery.* New York: Basic Books.

McCann, I. L. & Pearlman, L. A. (1990), Vicarious traumatization: A framework for understanding the psychological effects of working with victims. *J. Traumatic Stress,* 3:131–150.

Pearlman, L. A. & Saakvitne, K. (1995), *Trauma and the Therapist.* New York: Norton.

9 Disease, Death, and Group Process from a Psychodynamic Point of View

Barbara K. Eisold

Groups for people with AIDS have been run by leaders whose orientations and experience vary widely; a great deal has been written on the subject (Anderson, Laudry, and Kerby, 1991). The object of this chapter is to describe one such group, which was guided as much by my own particular interest in understanding the complexity of member experience as it was to provide "support." As a clinician now for some years, I have been surprised to discover that my interest in my chosen field is sustained as much by a kind of passion to understand as it is by a wish to help. This "passion" is the moving force behind psychoanalysis. Not all psychoanalysts want to understand for the same reasons, however. I work on the premise that if I can comprehend the implications of experience at each phase of development, I will always be able to accommodate the difficulties, even those with the most dire consequences, including those ending in death. This premise, needless to say, is something of a fantasy: one cannot always easily grasp the full implications of human experience, *especially* when death is the sting. In fact, cumulative loss cannot be very well accommodated; I learned this from running my group. Before I began, all I knew was that people by the thousands were dying of AIDS, and I felt compelled to better understand what they were going through, having had little firsthand experience with death myself. The Gay Men's Health Crisis (GMHC) in New York City, I knew, was doing the most comprehensive job of any agency at the time (1988) in providing service to its clients. Hence, with no idea of what I was getting into, I signed on to lead a group there, as one of approximately 90 volunteer clinicians. A few weeks later I had completed the required orientation and was ready to start.

The Group

Choosing Members

In those days at GMHC, the prospective group leader had to commit herself for a year, whereas each member promised only 12 weeks. Each group met weekly at GMHC, for 90 minutes at a time. Because I planned to run my group alone (which I did for two of my three years' work there), I chose to meet during the workday, rather than in the evening or on weekends, because this was convenient for me. Without fully realizing it, in this way I set up a situation in which the only men available to attend my group were those already not working (and on disability), or those independently employed and able to set their own hours.

In order to begin, I made a series of appointments to meet prospective members individually, almost always at my private office. Interviews, which lasted from 40 to 60 minutes, inevitably began easily; the man would describe the history of his diagnosis, an event which, for any person with HIV disease, is a traumatic experience. In addition, I wanted to know something about the man's living conditions. Specifically I wanted to know about: (1) his interpersonal support system, such as whether he lived alone or with others, how robust his network of friends was, whether his family knew of his HIV status and their reaction to it; (2) the physical layout at his home, especially in regard to the accessibility of the street from his apartment; and (3) whether or not he had a doctor he liked. I wanted to have a sense of who each man was and how much "support" he might need from the group and from me. Of course, in answering these questions, the man inevitably told me a great deal about himself. Often tears were shed. As I gained experience and interviewed new people, to replace those who had died, I learned to listen more carefully than I had at the beginning when the prospective member described his relationships with various medical personnel. I learned that the way in which the man had gone about obtaining help with his illness was indicative of how committed he was to fighting it and, therefore, how unambivalent he was about wanting to live.

At his interview, nearly every prospective member asked what the group would be like. At the beginning I said I did not know exactly, never having led one like it before. I said that the group would have to define its own goals. When asked, as I frequently was, why I had chosen to lead the prospective group, I said that I had had little personal experience of death, that I felt compelled by the AIDS crisis to do something to help, that I was deeply moved by people who seemed to be living quite dignified lives with the disease, and that I wanted to understand what the parameters of the experience were for these people.

The question concerning my reasons for wanting to run the group was the first of many that group members asked me about myself as the group progressed. I generally answered briefly, as honestly as I could. From the very beginning of this work, in fact, I felt strongly that it was "right" to answer questions about myself when they were asked; whatever each question might mean to the asking person (and certainly we could discuss that), I did not know how much time there would be to "play" with the projections that it might contain. In addition, withholding simple information about myself seemed unfair. Because I wanted to learn intimate details about the most final and most serious experience of their lives, I thought I had no "right" not to reveal simple information about myself. An attitude of openness on my part was therefore apparent from the first.

At the end of his interview, each man was told the day and time of the first group meeting. Most of the men who came to be interviewed agreed to become members. Those who did not (two or three of the ten or twelve I interviewed decided not to attend) said that they did not want to talk openly about themselves in a group, or that they wanted a group that would provide medically related information only. One politely said he was unable to arrange his work life to accommodate a daytime schedule.

The group began, after four or five weeks of interviews, in January of 1988, with nine members; they were between the ages of 21 and 45. Only one was from New York originally; six other states were represented. Four were born Catholic, two Jewish, three Protestant. All members were college graduates, all were white. (Although later there were men of color, originally only white men were on the list I was given.)

Some had been or still were involved in the theater. The group also included a lawyer, a former stock market analyst, and an artist. One man did not seem to have done much of anything; I characterized him to myself as a drifter. Later we had academics, a librarian, teachers, and advertising men.

Early Definition of Group Purpose

At the beginning, in part because of the relative homogeneity of its membership (Tunnell, 1991), things went easily in my group. I had had enough previous experience as a leader to know that groups are most successful when members define both the subject matter they want to discuss and the ground rules they want to follow. When things seemed to bog down, guided by the wish to understand, I thought I would ask questions. At the beginning, however, I did not have to do much questioning. Spontaneously, members began by taking turns telling how and when they had been diagnosed and how their lovers (if they had them) and their families had reacted. Within and between there was some discussion of medical protocols and medical expertise. This took some weeks and bonded members to one another in an upbeat way. A list of members' addresses and telephone numbers was circulated. Rules were made about beginning and ending on time. It was agreed, however, that death was not to be discussed. No one believed it would happen to him, I think. Nor did any man, at that point, want to go deeply into his feelings about the meaning of the disease to him. Hope is what each man wanted to sustain, and to that end "support" is what every man said he wanted.

Certainly "support" was an important component of what the group provided. Above all, this support mitigated the profound isolation that many felt with the disease. It also created a background against which men helped one another construct a kind of optimistic outlook, one in which disease and death could be denied in a fashion that was probably quite healthy (Tunnell, 1991). When I asked questions about this, I was told that discussion of death would be "stressful," and "stress" was to be avoided at all costs because it was known to create vulnerability to disease. In contrast, discussion of medical protocols was not "stressful." Indeed, periodically this took up so much of our time that I questioned its value and, because the medical discussions were often quite dull, the group agreed to keep them to a minimum and to advise each other, if necessary, outside of the 90-minute meetings. Some members began to socialize with one another and to use each other's professional expertise between meetings. Things went on this way until the first death.

The First Death

Inevitably, the first death in a group is a turning point (Tunnell, 1991; Gabriel, 1991). In my group, the fact that it occurred only four months after we began probably heightened its impact. In fact, it came as a complete surprise. James, the member who died, was the man I have described as something of a drifter. He had not been taking AZT, which at the time was the best treatment available as a deterrent of HIV disease, and had chosen homeopathic rather than conventional medical care. He was receiving this care from a "doctor" who did not appear to have any hospital affiliation.

James had been ill and was absent from the group for two or three weeks, during which time I had been calling his house on a regular basis to ask after his health. I did this in part so that I could report to the group about him, because it very soon became obvious that group members did not much want to call him themselves. When asked about this, they said they were afraid to "get involved": it would be "too stressful." In addition, they wanted to deny the seriousness of James's illness and, by implication, the seriousness of their own. If they made contact with him by telephone, their denial would be challenged. At the same time, they did not want to forget him; whenever I said that I had been in touch with his roommate, they wanted to hear every detail. Because of this conflict in them, I took on the role of information gatherer and message carrier from the very start. It became my job, so to speak, to know as much as I could about the circumstances surrounding each man's illness and, eventually, each man's death, and to report to the remaining group members as fully as I could. They always listened carefully to everything I had to say. Often, as was the case with the first death, what they heard made them angry. Death itself infuriated them. As much as they mourned each loss (and wanted to remember the dead man in detail), they also got irritated at anyone who died. To them it seemed a kind of betrayal.

This state of mind was especially prevalent in the first months of group meetings. Angry as they were about the death of a man, they seemed to want all the information I could supply about how it happened in order to learn, from the dead man's mistakes, how to defend themselves more effectively against dying. The first death was perhaps the one we all learned the most from in this regard, because its rapidity was more the result of bad management than of the actual disease status of its victim.

As a result of my telephone calls to his home, I had developed something of a relationship with James's roommate, who had not been close to James, it appeared; he had been thrust into the role of guardian, nevertheless, almost against his will. In fact, without trying very hard, I had become something of a consultant to this roommate, who was quite isolated and desperate himself because of the responsibilities that had inadvertently come his way. The roommate was a man who believed in conventional medical care for PWAs (People With AIDS) and he, along with others among James's friends, had tried to procure this for James. But James, irritable and feverish as he was, had turned them down. Meanwhile, one afternoon while the roommate was out, James's homeopathic acquaintances kidnapped him and took him to Long Island, to a talented healer friend, a woman who they believed could cure him. She took one look at him and would not let him in her house; she immediately called an ambulance and had him carted off to a small, overcrowded, local hospital where they had very little experience treating PWAs. He died that night, in a hall where the hospital staff had left him, unattended and alone. His roommate, completely unprepared as he had been, both for the severity of James's illness and the feud with his friends, felt guilty and terrible about this death and blamed himself.

My group ruminated over this story for some time. They were appalled. The need for a good doctor with solid hospital connections was clear from this tale: one's life could be saved by such a person. The need, in addition, for a reliable support system of friends, people one knew well and whom one trusted, also became clear, for it was obvious that failure in this regard had let James down. The flaws in James's character, which had brought on the havoc that contributed to his rapid demise, were discussed at great length. Obviously, they concluded, one dies as one lives. The group felt sorry that they had not understood James sooner. They believed that if they had, they might have been able to do more for him.

In this way, not only did disease and death enter our presence in no uncertain terms, but it also seemed advisable that we get to know one another more intimately. In that way, it was surmised, perhaps death could be retarded. Thus James's death became a cautionary tale.

The Role of the Group Leader

The first death was a turning point, not only for the group, but for me as its leader. I very quickly discovered that I was not going to be able to resist the compelling need to find out as much as I could about each member's situation when he became ill. As I have said, the pressure I felt on this score was partly induced by the need of group members to "know," despite their fear of the effect that "knowing" might have on them. As their leader, I was not aware enough to pick up on this conflict and question it with them, perhaps because I was blinded by my own need to understand. Instead, I accepted the role I seemed to have been assigned, perhaps because it appealed to me. Being authorized to ask questions in order to understand, and then to provide my group with information, made me feel less helpless than I might have felt had I too been in the dark about each member's disease status and health-care system. In doing this, I felt as if I had been given a clear and important role to play. As a consequence, unlike other group leaders (see Gabriel, 1991), I not only had no trouble discussing the first death when it happened, but as other members got sicker, I found myself making hospital and home visits as frequently as I could, ostensibly to learn as much as I could about them. When I could not visit, I telephoned.

In retrospect, I was not at all prepared for what occurred once hospital and home visits began. First of all, in doing this I became something of a consultant to the families and friends of group members and, in one hospital, to some of the nursing staff as well. In other cases, when members were able to attend the group almost to the end, I got very attuned to the point at which the final illness was about to happen (a certain restlessness seemed to take them over) and, once or twice, when they lived alone, I invited myself to their homes in order to help them arrange hospitalization for what we both knew would be the last time.

In still other situations, I became aware when visiting that some men seemed to need to show their bodies to me and to other people as well. One very appealing young man, for example, lay uncovered in his hospital bed, clothed only in his undershorts. He was, in fact, so appealing that many people sympathetically touched his feet in passing, until finally these pats caused an infection. Another man displayed to all his visitors the apparatus for urination attached to his bed and regularly gave demonstrations of how it worked. A third waited until company was present to give himself the injections he required. A fourth, very ill but living at home, spent evenings in various bars when he could. There he would throw his shirt off displaying his Hickman catheter, along with his naked chest, for all to see. His greatest wish, he said, was to be photographed life-size, catheter and all, and displayed this way in bus-stop advertisements, behind glass. A very articulate man, he explained to me his conviction that if he could exist as a whole person in the eyes of others, in spite of his injury, he might, in turn, regain a sense of his own integrity and extend his life. Through him I was made aware, for the first time, of the restorative function that self-display has for some people when they feel that their personal integrity is threatened.[1]

In all of this I was presented with a clinical role that was different

1. Stolorow (1975), a self psychologist interested in the self-esteem-regulating

from anything I had ever before undertaken. I was captivated as much by the excitement of its newness as by the fact that I seemed able to do the work. I was also profoundly moved by what I saw and touched beyond words with the closeness I was allowed to share. I thought then and still think that the work was a great privilege. It was certainly an antidote to any feeling of helplessness I might have had. Unlike many who work with PWAs (see Winiarski, 1991, for example), my own helplessness in contending with the disease was rarely on my mind.

In a bimonthly supervision group at GMHC I discovered that clinicians varied widely when it came to making home and hospital visits. Some went regularly, as I did, others never went at all. All points of view on this subject were accepted and discussed, along with the potential for burnout. This made it easy for me not to question the compulsion I felt to make visits. In retrospect, I wish I had done a little more questioning, in part because of the group dynamic it now seemed to have represented. My men, as I have said, were afraid to have much close contact with one another when they were gravely ill, for fear they themselves might catch something. I accepted this fear. I did not question its exaggerated nature, evidenced by the fact that they rarely even called each other on the telephone when they were ill. At the same time, I accepted the role of information collector without questioning myself. In retrospect, greater understanding of this dynamic might have been useful to all. At the least, it might have led to a more detailed and useful understanding of the need for denial.

Soon after beginning my group, I joined a monthly supervision group run by Yvonne Agazarian (1989) and, in addition, attended weekend-long workshops she directed twice yearly. Ostensibly, all of this was to learn more about group dynamics. I did learn quite a bit, in fact. Among other things, Agazarian teaches a subgrouping technique that mitigates scapegoating. It works as follows: whenever a member expresses a new or possibly controversial opinion, he is advised by the leader to find others who agree with him. The search not only turns the attention of members away from immediate argument, it often ends in members forming partnerships of sorts with one another. In this fashion, no one is left too long feeling isolated because of something he has said, and no one can be scapegoated.

Agazarian's subgrouping technique was a useful tool. In addition,

---

aspects of what he calls "narcissism," reviews the topic of self-display in terms of its reparative function. Although at times the ways in which the self is displayed may be difficult to witness (as was true for me in the case of the man in my group who gave himself injections in my presence) and may contain other elements (perhaps a wish to inflict suffering on others), the essential function of the self-display as reparative seems undeniable to me. See Petrucelli in this volume for a similar clinical example.

this supervision gave me the opportunity to listen to other people's tales about non-AIDS-related groups. It gave me the opportunity to think about the effect of group dynamics in general. But above all, it was immensely supportive, perhaps because I was the only one among Agazarian's supervisees who was leading a group in which members were dying of AIDS. In my supervision group at GMHC, by contrast, everyone was leading such a group, and there was quite a bit of unaddressed judgment and competition about who was doing this in the most "healthy" way. In Agazarian's supervision group, because there was not quite this kind of competition, I felt greater freedom to address issues that were purely related to group dynamics.

Members' Experiences: Life on Fast-Forward versus Despair

As the group developed, surprising changes seemed to occur in the lives of some members. These changes, described as well by others in regard to PWAs (Nichols, 1986; Beckett and Rutan, 1990; Sleek, 1996), seemed to imply a deeper, more creative commitment to life; they seemed as much a surprise to members themselves as to me. For example, one man, an artist who made his living by selling hand-painted glass plates to elegant department stores in New York City, began painting bird people on glass instead. He had done this before, but under the impact of HIV disease he began turning them out at a rapid pace. He showed them at a local gallery. These extraordinary figures—wonderfully pastoral, often very powerful, always slightly flawed self-representations—began to sell like hotcakes. Their creator began earning more money than he had ever earned in his life, which he vastly enjoyed. He also developed a very complex relationship with his female assistant, a closer relationship than he had ever had with anyone. He discussed this at length with the group.

A second man, who was very young, began to write for the first time in his life. Before he died, he had completed two short stories and the outline for a novel. These works were given to me to critique; they bound him to me in a way he hoped might extend his life, he said. A third man cooperated on a book, written under church auspices; it was a collection of stories by people with various life-threatening illnesses, whose lives had been "transformed" by disease. A fourth man apprenticed himself to a well-known healer who began using his services to assist her with her clients. A fifth man created a radio show of his own. Two people bought country houses with their lovers and planted gardens. Gardens were discussed at great length in the group. Everyone seemed to know something about them. For a short time the creative outpouring was big and full of joy. As one man put it, tongue-in-cheek, he could hardly thank the disease enough for what it had done for him. It was as if these potentially very creative people were living their lives on fast-forward, trying to get done as much as they could before death. The struggle, the bitter potential of death, was always with them, but the energy they had to begin things was the energy of youth, of people who have not given up and who do not feel their lives have been lived for naught.[2]

Death, no longer so completely denied, began to occupy a special place among us. Some people had definite ideas about who or what death looked like. We had occasional discussions about how it (he, she) appeared to them. Some people visualized him as a snake, a mad dog, a shadow beneath the eye. Two men dreamt regularly about wrestling with him and surviving the fight. One man died in his dream and after death came out, surprisingly, to the same world he had left behind! Psychiatrists Spiegel and Yalom (1978) describe this kind of discussion as routine in groups of cancer patients that they ran for years.

Fears about becoming gravely ill and helpless also came up for discussion. Everyone dreaded having to depend on others for help. Funeral arrangements were on every member's mind. In addition, there were constant worries about relatives left behind. Some members were more able to discuss these topics than others. Some did better with them when they were visited in the hospital or at home.

For many (but not all) members, a review of their lives seemed necessary before they could become creatively engaged. Inevitably, this included some review of their feelings about growing up gay. We heard about men ruthlessly teased by peers all through childhood and

---

2. Kohut (1977) describes a kind of "guiltless despair" observed in some people, in late middle age, when they "discover that the basic patterns of their self . . . have not been realized" (p. 271) and cannot remedy this situation in the time and with the energies at their disposal.

In contrast, Richard Sterba (1990), a very productive psychoanalyst who felt neither guilt nor despair about the life he had lived, reported a dream, following a major heart attack, that occurred as he was considering two new projects, shortly before he died: "I was on an ocean liner. I found two dead flies on the deck. . . . Deciding that I had to bury them at sea, I folded a piece of writing paper to make two coffins, paper that was unusually large, like the ones I recall Freud using for his manuscripts. I set the two paper coffins on the water; a large wave carried them out to sea" (p. 110). In part because of this dream, he realized that he could not complete the two new projects. His energy for such projects was gone. Without despair, however, he could give them up, set them out to sea.

I read these as examples of what elderly people sometimes feel—as they face death. There is a striking difference, however, between each of these feeling states and the feeling states of the men in my AIDS group. My experience of most of the men in my group was that a surprising amount of energy—perhaps fueled by hope or the wish not to miss out on their desserts—took hold of them and pressed them into service. As exemplified above, the elderly, whether despairing or not, do not seem to have such energy at their disposal.

adolescence for not being "manly" enough; about extraordinary abuse at the hands of fathers, uncles, or brothers; about a boy who mourned the day he outgrew his mother's shoes; about a family in which *all* the siblings were gay and were also bonded against parents who hated them for it; about a mother whose anger at discovering her son's homosexuality had separated them for years. No two stories were the same. Some included years of drug and alcohol abuse; many members were graduates of AA, NA, or GA. A great deal of time, in fact, was spent on guilt and the idea that AIDS was payment for "bad" behavior. "Badness" was often linked with "gayness" and AIDS in their minds, as well as with substance abuse and other extremes of behavior.[3] Members were extraordinarily respectful and helpful to one another in contending with the intense feelings that were raised by these issues.

Then there were those in whom bitterness or despair seemed to have lodged permanently. Among these men, group attendance often did not last for more than a few months, despite considerable effort on my part to engage them. More of these joined the group later, taking the places of those original members who had died. These were sometimes people (as James had been) who had never been able to get a foothold anywhere in life. Often they were still abusing alcohol or drugs. Sometimes they were men who had lived their professional lives within a structure in which they did not have to think about what to do. Left by the disease without that structure, they were often at greater risk for depression than those who had always lived more independent working lives and knew how to stay occupied and engaged. Often these despairing men were also unable to let anyone help them, not being accustomed to closeness of any kind. For these men, my group was probably of little help. There was not enough time to ameliorate their depression.

Rage

Any disabling disease creates rage in those who suffer from it, because of the helplessness it engenders, and the patience required for its

3. My experience in work with all sorts of people who are HIV-positive is that "badness" is generally connected to whatever it is they did that gave them the disease. If the disease was contracted from intravenous drug use, they think of themselves as "bad" for having used drugs. If, in the case of many women, the disease was contracted through out-of-wedlock sexual contact, *that* is considered "bad." It is the very rare person indeed who, having become the victim of a terrible disease, does not try to blame him- or herself for having it. Self-blame often seems the most immediate way to combat feelings of helplessness. It is easier to accept the idea that one has sinned and believe that atonement will rectify things than it is to accept a disastrous situation in which one is convinced nothing can be done.

management. People with AIDS are, in addition, faced with their minority status, their fear of abandonment on this account, the paucity of medical information available, and the fear of contagion the disease creates in others. On this last, most painful score, group members routinely shared stories about how they had not been invited to one family gathering or another because their relatives feared that children would become infected. They told a medley of other stories as well: of friends who surreptitiously sterilized dishes, cleaning ladies who quit, subway personnel who questioned their half-fare status, doctors and dentists who refused to serve them, stories in which their surprise, hurt, and anger resonated.

Some men got so angry at the disease and what it represented to them that the anger itself became a motive for living, husbanding resources, fighting, screaming. There was one gentle, outwardly complacent, uneducated black man from Brooklyn—bisexual, ex-alcoholic, with a large family. He was a late-comer to the group (he entered at the beginning of my third year, just after I had been joined by a co-leader) and was accustomed to attending groups. He was an old hand at Alcoholics Anonymous, and actually belonged to two AA groups in Brooklyn. He was hooked on *group*, so to speak. He was also just beginning to have grandchildren. His groups, his family, his burgeoning wish to have faith in God, and a streak of stubborn determination, fueled by frustration and rage, kept him motivated to live for some time. He was simply unwilling to miss the joy of his recent reconciliation with his daughter and of observing the changes each day in his new grandson, with whom he was living at that time. Thus, as his symptoms increased, he struggled more and more with his God, because this God, he thought, threatened to deny him life. Having relinquished his major "sins," alcohol and promiscuity, some time ago, he thought he deserved better treatment. His rage at God and the disease motivated him to use his good intelligence to search for the best medical care he could get, which, indeed, he got, in spite of his lack of education and his other so-called disadvantages. I know this because I kept in touch with him by telephone long after he stopped attending my group.

The deepest vein of rage emerged from the humiliation some group members experienced as their symptoms increased. Two or three times, this rage exploded in the group, propelling the affected member out, never to return again. Others (Nichols, 1986; Beckett and Rutan, 1990; Tunnell, 1991) have also described rage as the route chosen by some to leave an AIDS group when worsening symptoms are experienced as demeaning.

The clearest example of this in my own group resulted from a fight that erupted between the lawyer, our most articulate, best-educated member, a man of huge physical stature, and the aforementioned radio commentator, a short, diminutive man. The lawyer had been diagnosed with AIDS, the commentator with ARC (AIDS-related complex). In those days, people with ARC were thought to live longer than people with AIDS, and for all intents and purposes, the man with ARC seemed to be doing quite well. I do not remember what precipitated their fight. Indeed, the larger man had seemed so angry in the previous weeks that I myself had found him frightening; I had actually consulted with a colleague about him. On that particular day, the smaller man must have said something unpleasant, if not actually insulting, about the characteristics of the boastful, periodically hostile, bigger man. Suddenly the latter was on his feet, screaming invectives at the little man. This lasted for some moments until, with a powerful thrust, the big man picked up the pillow he had brought to sit on, threw it in the little man's face, and then stormed out.

A long moment of silence went by. No one ran out of the room to fetch the big man back (we worked hard to understand this later, for apparently he had waited some minutes outside for someone to do just this) and, perhaps because of this, he was forever gone. None of our telephone attempts to secure his return succeeded. Soon after this, he moved to the Florida Keys, where the symptoms that had already begun before he left (and were the reason he was sitting on a pillow) became very grave. I kept in occasional touch with him by telephone. Other group members called him as well, for he had been very important to them all. Nearly a year later, he returned for one last visit, and then he died. As for the man with ARC, he too left the group after that terrible day. Nothing I could do would bring him back.

Once or twice I was the target of a member's rage. I was, after all, the only person in the group whose life was not in danger from the disease. When the subject of rage and resentment toward me was raised (I tried to bring it up on a regular basis), the majority of members agreed that they could not afford to be angry at me, because I had the task of remembering them when they were gone. Nevertheless, some were obviously furious at me. Periodically I got accused of being grossly unfair or homophobic. Often, when this happened, the man who made the accusation left in a huff, never to be seen again. The telephone call that followed, asking him to return at least for one final session, never succeeded. This behavior—the rapid disappearance of a man after making accusations—made me think that one function of his rage was to make separation quick and relatively painless. But while it was happening, I felt completely at a loss as to what to do, and I sometimes felt angry and hurt as well. I used my supervision groups to help me contend with these feelings.

Countertransference

Describing my reaction to the rage of group members leads me directly to the subject of countertransference, which I want to discuss in regard to sexual orientation on the one hand, and to disease and death on the other.

Sexual Orientation

When I began my AIDS group I had not given the subject of sexual orientation very much thought and, as a result, did not hold any definite position on the subject. The men in my group, therefore, may have experienced shifts in my opinions as the subject was discussed. I was also hungry for information; I wanted to understand the developmental implications of differences in this regard, if indeed there are any. In fact, the group contributed to my wish for this kind of information because so many of its members were themselves so pained by their own developmental histories.

Motivated by my own curiosity, I worked hard to learn. During one year at GMHC I also completed a miniresidency at Mt. Sinai Hospital, in New York, in human sexuality. Later I taught an undergraduate course on the subject at New York University. More recently I have had as patients two young children, the sons of gay men. The delineation of gender-role-related behaviors became a central part of our work together because of its importance to them. Thus I have been able to observe firsthand something of the way in which children position themselves differently, early in life, in regard to these issues (Eisold, in press). It seems to me now that the process of developing erotic taste, or what the psychoanalyst Ethel Person (1980) calls a "sex print," is not something we know much about. Certainly, we are in no position now to make any generalizations about the relationship between this and other identifications that evolve during early development.

Understanding much more clearly now how little we know about issues related to sex and gender has made the subject matter seem less compelling than it did earlier. These days my urgent questions seem to be about other things.

Disease and Death

The feelings I experienced about disease and death during the years I ran my group were often unexpected and irrational. Others (Kübler-Ross, 1969; Sontag, 1978) have remarked on the way in which this can happen to both patient and caregiver when together they are living with a fatal illness. Irrationalities also multiply when the disease in question is sexually transmissible, as Santorelli (1988) and Winiarski (1991) both describe.

Although anger and helplessness are common to this experience, in fact I frequently felt a kind of feverish joy in working with the men in my group, pulled as I was by the poignancy of their situation. Later I recovered, in my own reanalysis, an early experience of near drowning,[4] which might have had something to do with this "pull." But I was unaware of this at the time, and other things instead presented themselves as compelling.

First of all, perceiving the aliveness of so many men and seeing its creative results had surprising effects on me. Frequently I felt close to a very vital source. At times this closeness seemed a bit dangerous. My dreams during these periods, full of my own fantasied HIV symptoms, reflected this danger. At still other times, boundaries seemed entirely unclear. For example, I experienced one man as having stepped over my outer boundaries without my knowledge. After he died, it seemed to me that he had managed to get further inside the wall of my defenses than I habitually let anyone. About another, I felt at times that no boundaries existed at all between us and that it was my vitality the man was using to get through his day. With a third, I felt periodically that his rage would demolish me. With many men I did not feel anywhere near this degree of connection. The artist who painted on glass was one of these. In spite of my much cooler feelings for him, however, I did get to know his social world very well (mother, nurses, friends), and he continued to be a most devoted group member until his death.

Although I tried to be equally available to all members, I did not succeed. I did not much question myself about the effects of this discrepancy at the time. I was surprised and pleased that I could do the work at all, that I did not want to flee when men got sick, or even when they died. I had the illusion once in a while that I had a special relationship with death, that I knew death well, that we were friends. I understood for the first time then, that I had always had some kind of relationship with death, that "he" had always existed somewhere, on the left, in my mind's eye, as a sort of shadow. During the time I ran my group, "he" seemed to move closer, in this way altering my internal sense of the amount of time I myself have left to live.

---

4. At eighteen months of age, I fell into a swimming pool and nearly drowned. By sheer chance, I was pulled unconscious out of the water by a passing adolescent. Although I had been told about this experience I had no recollection of it until recently when, during a second analysis, it seemed to come back quite intensely. When this happened, it occurred to me that the "pull" I experienced toward PWAs was possibly motivated by the need to know better my own close shave with death.

By the beginning of the third year, many of the original group members had died. I was quite conscientious about mourning them, not only with those who remained, but alone. I went to as many funerals as I could and cried often. I often wrote things down about each man for the sake of my own well-being. I was frankly afraid of what effect *not* mourning might have on me. Nevertheless, my passion for the work began to wane. At the beginning of the third year, GMHC gave me a co-leader, someone I liked but had not known before. We replaced members, interviewing people together. The list of available clients had begun to diminish by then, however, and it became more and more difficult to get new members. I found the task increasingly arduous, in part, I think, because I wanted the old members back. Cumulative loss, even when people are individually mourned, has a numbing effect on the capacity to reconnect. As for the meetings themselves, sometimes only two men would show up for sessions, sometimes only one; four was the average. Surprisingly, the new men seemed colorless and uncompelling to me. Thus, with supervisory support, I gradually made the decision to leave, feeling that for myself and for the sake of new group members, it was time. I was no longer doing good work with them. I left with a feeling of gratitude. It is rare to have known so many extraordinary men.

References

Agazarian, Y. M. (1989), Group-as-a-whole systems theory and practice. *Group: J. Eastern Group Psychother. Soc.*, 13:3 & 4.

Anderson, J. B., Laudry, C. P. & Kerby, J. L. (1991), *AIDS Abstracts of the Psychological and Behavioral Literature*, 3rd ed. Washington, DC: American Psychological Association.

Beckett, A. & Rutan, J. S. (1990), Treating persons with ARC and AIDS in group psychotherapy. *Internat. J. Group Psychother.*, 40:19–29.

Eisold, B. K. (in press), Recreating mother: The consolidation of heterosexual gender identification in the young son of homosexual men: A clinical presentation. *J. Amer. Orthopsychiat. Assn.*

Gabriel, M. A. (1991), Group therapists' countertransference reactions to multiple deaths from AIDS. *Clin. Soc. Work*, 19:279–292.

Kohut, H. (1977), *The Restoration of the Self.* New York: International Universities Press.

Kübler-Ross, E. (1969), *On Death and Dying.* London: Macmillan.

Nichols, S. E. (1986), Psychotherapy and AIDS. In: *Contemporary Perspectives on Psychotherapy with Lesbians and Gay Men*, ed. T. S. Stein & C. J. Cohen. New York: Plenum, pp. 209–239.

Person, E. S. (1980), Sexuality as the mainstay of identity. In: *Women, Sex and Sexuality,* ed. C. R. Stimson & E. S. Person. Chicago, IL: University of Chicago Press.

Santorelli, M. (1988), Psychotherapeutic treatment of AIDS patients: Mental health perspectives. Unpublished doctoral dissertation, Yeshiva University.

Sleek, S. (1996), AIDS therapy: Patchwork of pain and hope. *APA Monitor,* 27, 6:1, 31.

Sontag, S. (1978), *Illness as Metaphor.* New York: Farrar, Straus.

Spiegel, D. & Yalom, I. D. (1978), A support group for dying patients. *Internat. J. Group Psychother.,* 28:233–245.

Sterba, R. F. (1990), Analysis without apparent resistance. *Internat. J. Psycho-Anal.,* 71:107–111.

Stolorow, R. D. (1975), Towards a functional view of narcissism. *Internat. J. Psycho-Anal.,* 56:179–185.

Tunnell, G. (1991), Complications in group psychotherapy with AIDS patients. *Internat. J. Group Psychother.,* 41:481–498.

Winiarski, M. G. (1991), *AIDS-Related Psychotherapy.* New York: Pergamon.

10 When a Patient Becomes HIV-Positive During Psychotherapy

Ernesto Mujica

Few today are ignorant of the gravity of HIV infection and the importance of safer sex practices. Exposing oneself to the risk of HIV infection, however, is often not simply suicidal, impulsive behavior. Because of its primary mode of transmission, namely, through the exchange of body fluids, HIV infection is a physiological process that is immersed in, and configured by, the personal and social influences that shape our modes of intimate contact with others. High-risk behavior or actual infection with HIV often has deeply personal and dynamic meanings. When explored therapeutically, these meanings can be uncovered, thereby expanding the patient's self-knowledge and curiosity about him- or herself, while aiding in the reduction of self-destructive patterns. Factors such as desire for intimacy, fear of aloneness or rejection, and low self-esteem, as well as one's sense of social integration versus isolation, are crucial.

Fantasies of becoming HIV-positive may develop at times of desperate isolation. This may be particularly true for those who have already lost persons dear to them through AIDS. Idealizing fantasies can offer one a hope of instant transformation; they can engender feelings of belonging and promise human contact and caring. Recently, to my initial surprise, this wish was expressed by a patient, a young gay man who experienced familial and social discrimination against his homosexuality combined with loss of employment. He expressed his fantasy of being HIV-positive as a way of finding longed-for comfort and caring. Within his idealized fantasy, once he became positive he would no longer be alone, he would become part of an important, socially acknowledged and definable group, with access to a network of support systems in an otherwise unconcerned and rejecting world.

For an HIV-negative person whose spouse or lover has tested positive, increased risk-taking behavior may express intense longings to reaffirm commitment to the partner, and may be triggered by anticipated feelings of loss and mourning. It is also important to consider those who have previously had the experience of distancing themselves from an HIV-positive lover or friend. Conscious as well as unconscious attempts at reparation with a previously rejected loved object, or guilt as a survivor, can be reflected through decreased attention to safer sex practices with new partners who may be HIV-positive.

High-risk behavior may also be evoked as a sudden, counterdepressive reaction following loss or separation from a partner who is HIV-positive. The daily restrictions and cautions that are entailed in securing low-risk behavior when partners are HIV-discordant can be suddenly lifted following a breakup of the relationship, or following the mourning period of a deceased partner, with the fantasied relief that one is no longer at risk. While these experiences may not be frequent, they can and do predispose some patients to let go of the restrictions of safer sex practices. Hence, a powerful wish to escape the deadly threat of HIV infection can be fostered by the use of denial and dissociation, with ensuing self-immersion in blissful feelings and fantasies of youthfulness, sexual attractiveness, passion, and love.

This chapter concerns my work with James, who seroconverted a year and a half after entering three times a week psychoanalysis with me. James is a single, gay Hispanic man in his late 20s, of small stature and slight build. He is highly intelligent, was educated at an Ivy League school, and is well traveled. At the time of seeking treatment he was distraught about his difficulties with Scott, his boyfriend of three years. He also complained of being unfulfilled by his job as an office assistant and feeling stagnated in his occupational development. During the earlier part of his treatment with me, James tended to be boyish and cute, easily flirtatious in his manner. These qualities contributed to his feeling unmanly and to his expectation that he would not be taken seriously by others. At times the effect of his manner was endearing, yet initially it also contributed to my own difficulty with taking him seriously. James had some awareness of these issues, yet he often felt hopeless regarding his ability to be assertive. In a compensatory manner, James emphasized his good looks, affable social manner, and intelligence to aid him in feeling more powerful.

James is the younger of two sons born abroad to a formerly wealthy South American family following a collapse of their family business. They immigrated to the United States before his first birthday. For most of his childhood his parents were still adapting to the traumatic changes that resulted from their separation from family and friends, as well as to their severe economic downfall. The family had had a chauffeur, cook, and nanny. His brother, who is 10 years older than James, had attended a prestigious private school in South America and had dressed in the finest tailored clothing. Upon their arrival in the United States, and throughout his latency years, they lived in a working-class suburb of a large northeastern city; his father worked full-time and simultaneously studied to reestablish his business degree. The dramatically different socioeconomic context of his early childhood contributed to his feeling deprived and left out, alienated from his family.

During James's first year of life, his mother reportedly sat for long hours, day after day, crying, with her newborn child in her arms, deeply depressed about their multiple losses. As a child, James states, he was often hit with a belt by his parents, particularly by his mother. "She used to hit me and chase me around the house; it was very frightening. I remember until I was about nine, she'd chase me around the house like a lunatic. I've told her I'll never forgive her for it. I think she couldn't stand not controlling me. I was very imaginative. I did a lot of shows and things with other kids. To my parents it was all a headache."

His memories about his relationships with peers during his early childhood are often good ones. He was popular among his friends and was often the leader of the pack. At that time, in contrast to his adolescence, he recalls feeling tough and able to fend for himself in his peer group. However, this did not parallel his relationship with his older brother, whom he described as often physically and verbally abusive from early on. The impact of intense fraternal conflict on his difficulties in self-assertiveness as an adult, as well as on his tendency to become involved with controlling and emotionally distant men, has been a key topic of discussion in his treatment. He describes that when he was approximately seven years old, his brother would hit him repeatedly, then kiss him "all over my face while holding me down when I started crying. . . . I used to be so afraid of him, all he had to do was raise his hand and I'd be covering my face in a panic, terrified." The erotic components of mild physical threat with male lovers became an important theme in our work.

During his early adolescence, James's father had become economically successful, and they were able to buy a home in an upper-middle-class neighborhood. Paradoxically, the higher economic and educational benefits that were now available to James precipitated a marked descent in his social status relative to his new peers. Furthermore, he experienced an abrupt and painful separation from the friendships he had established in his working-class community. He had grown accustomed to the ethnically diverse children who had been his close friends during his early childhood. James was now confronted by wealthy non-Hispanic peers who were quick to reject and shame him for his differences. In contrast, his brother and parents assimilated with confidence and familiarity in their new, wealthier environment, as they felt restored to their affluent origins.

During this transition period, James also became increasingly aware of his developing sexual attraction toward other boys, which further promoted his sense of being different from his peers. His self-consciousness added to his being perceived as queer, which, in fact, gradually brought an onslaught of epithets from his classmates: "sissy" and "spic" became common verbal assaults to endure. Though girls were often attracted to him, he wanted to be their friend rather than their boyfriend. In contrast, his brother had become very popular in his new school, and boasted of his many girlfriends. In the meantime, his parents avoided any recognition of James's developing homosexual orientation; in fact, his family's outright ridicule of homosexuals implicitly assured that they would not approve of his being gay.

As a young adult, James ventured to make a place for himself in a world that was largely unwelcoming by entering the more exotic, jet-set circles of the gay elite. Perhaps this was a form of what Frank Browning (1994) has referred to as a "journey of difference": "Because we do not recognize ourselves in the available popular plots, we are drawn—liking it or not—to probe further mysteries of fate and flesh" (p. 16). He sought the company of attractive, wealthy men and thrived on "fabulous" experiences. He felt protected from life's daily pains by the cushion of abundance and glamour, even if this cushion proved to be temporary. Because of his companions' wealth and, sporadically, his parents' indulgence, he sampled the latest chic restaurants and spent weekend vacations abroad. However, he often emerged frustrated or insulted from these ventures.

James wanted to be in treatment with a therapist who would accept his homosexual orientation. He described his previous therapist, whom he had seen for two years, as having interpreted his homosexuality as the result of his not feeling sufficiently masculine and powerful. James stated that his therapist felt he sought relationships with men as a way of taking in what he felt he lacked as a man, as well as a way of obtaining the care and sense of identity that he did not get from his relationship with his father. Though James stated he could understand the issues that were being "interpreted" by his therapist, he also felt that his sexual orientation was nonetheless homosexual, and he did not feel invested in seeking to change this fact. Despite his not feeling understood by his previous therapist in this important aspect, James did not challenge his therapist directly. Though he expressed a sense of disappointment, there was hardly a trace of anger expressed by James toward his previous therapist in this regard.

In contrast to James's relative passivity, I felt my own objections rise against the interpretations he had reportedly been given. These interpretations seemed stereotypical, aimed toward undoing his homosexual orientation and undermining his sense of self, uniqueness, and identity. I also thought to myself, however, that I was being moved by James toward taking the role of rescuer, and I felt concerned about his potential for remaining the perpetual victim. In addition, I had the sense that by getting others to be critical toward him (as had his previous therapist), he was vicariously identifying with their hostility and disapproval. I felt that his vicarious identification with his abusers expressed dissociated aspects of himself, perhaps reflecting his self-hatred for being dependent and submissive, different and queer.

What might I be unconsciously reenacting with James? In fantasy, perhaps I would help him feel he had found a sense of relatedness and belonging as a Hispanic man in the United States. Perhaps I would be able to help him recapture the well-being and emotional closeness he fantasied his brother had experienced with his parents prior to his birth. I was also a Hispanic immigrant as a young child. Perhaps in my own attempts to reassure myself that I had not lost all contact with my native language and culture, I wanted to help him achieve a stronger connection to his family's cultural origins. The fact that he was gay enhanced my experience of him as being unique and endangered, vulnerable to rejections from others as well as to his own bouts of self-loathing. In my own countertransference explorations, I envisioned him as a comrade in exile, and as a younger brother to protect and defend from the harshness and cruelty of others.

During our initial sessions, James sought to impress me with his ability to work with dream interpretations, and he let me know that his previous therapist was very impressed with his abilities in this respect.

At times his presentation of dreams felt like an offering, a lure for my attention. Simultaneously it represented a devaluation of his more immediate feelings and experiences, accompanied by the expressed fear that I would otherwise lose interest in him.

James had repeated experiences of being picked on and devalued by his boyfriend, Scott, paralleling his childhood abuse by his older brother. According to James, Scott often made fun of his ideas and plans about his career goals. He reported feeling that Scott was only interested in him because he was charming and attractive, an exciting sexual partner. James also constantly feared that Scott would leave him for a new lover.

The parallels between his relationship with Scott and his childhood longing for attention and acceptance from his rejecting older brother became increasingly clear. Unmasking these connections between his early object relations and his current difficulties in relationships often led to important, though painful, realizations. James gained mastery in his ability to explore his motivations and the various roles he played, especially as the seductive target of his lover's hostility. He came to recognize the hidden strengths he was afraid to unveil: his acute perception of unconscious motivations and weakness in others, his awareness of his own intellectual strengths, and his rarely used ability to be forcefully assertive.

Early on in our work I inquired about their HIV status, and James stated that he and Scott had both tested negative within the past year. When I inquired about their sexual practices, James stated they did not use condoms when having sex with each other, but that they were very careful to use condoms if either of them had sexual intercourse with a third person, which they sometimes did. James's initial tone during these discussions emphasized how strongly he felt about using condoms: "It would be really stupid to let anyone come inside without a condom, it would be suicidal." He was emphatic that Scott was well aware of safer sex practices, and that Scott had in fact run some workshops on safer sex practices and HIV. Yet, later within the same session, James said that he and Scott would go to sex clubs, and I asked, "At the club, have you allowed people to penetrate you without a condom?" He answered, "I did once, I was really drugged, I didn't really know what I was doing." He then reiterated that this had occurred many months ago and that he had recently tested negative once again.

We explored at length the effects of wearing a condom, which he objectively viewed as essential for protective reasons, yet subjectively experienced as an interference with "fusion," which seemed to represent intimacy and trust during intercourse. "Rubbers are antiseptic. To wear one, it feels like you're pushing the person away. When wearing a rubber, fusion isn't possible." I let him know that I was very concerned about his exposing himself to HIV infection, and that I felt he minimized the extent to which he continued to be at risk. He expressed feeling that it was very difficult to have to confront aspects of himself with me of which he felt ashamed. He acknowledged, of his own accord, that I helped him increase his self-awareness in a manner that was ultimately helpful; yet he was beginning to feel uncomfortably controlled by my vigilant concern.

Approximately six months after we had been working together, he reported, with a sense of cautious and mischievous excitement, that he had seen a wildlife television program concerning animals that are hunters and those that are their prey. At the time, we were in the midst of discussing his tendency to give up control in his relationships and to hand himself over, so to speak, when engaged with someone whom he perceived as stronger and more assertive than he. James explained that the wildlife film had shown a lion eating a zebra, and that he had experienced excitement and pleasure in viewing this, which had also disturbed him. "When I see the lion eating the zebra I don't see the pain. I see how it could be pleasurable to the zebra, it's weird, but it's also kind of sexual. What was pleasurable was the feeling of being devoured, like being wanted so much that someone could want to eat you alive, it's powerful, really carnal. Though I don't like to hurt anyone physically and don't like being hurt myself, it's a turn-on to have the fantasy of being brutalized by an authoritarian, powerful big man, being taken over; it's like being swallowed and eaten alive."

In my work with James, I have found it very useful to consider Jessica Benjamin's (1988) emphasis on "need for recognition" as the core of the masochist's unconscious desire:

> Longing for recognition lies beneath the sensationalism of power and powerlessness, that the unrecognizable forms often taken by our desire are the result of a complicated but ultimately understandable process—a process which explains how our deepest desires for freedom and communion become implicated in control and submission [p. 84].

We explored the theme of the lion and the zebra within the transference relationship. From this perspective, James experienced me as a coercive force, trying to rid him of his impulsive sexuality while fostering his desires to develop more emotionally stable, though less exciting, relationships. He also explored my role in devouring him. He was my object of study, and in this way, my object of desire. "I had a moment last night as I was falling asleep when I thought of you and of your becoming so close to me. I was anxious and nervous, almost scared in a shocking way, like you were entering my body somehow. I felt like you were devouring me, kind of, like the image of the lion and the zebra. I know you don't come with harm or hatred, but it's kind of frightening."

During a particularly fruitful session at the end of the first year of analysis, James described his experience of feeling that he had a porcelain doll within him, which he brought to the surface and experienced as a mask under specific circumstances: "With the porcelain doll side of me I seek to manipulate the other person with shallow things, like my looks. If someone is attracted to me when I'm that way I think, 'You fool, you fell for this, it's a fantasy, don't believe me, it's not me, it's an illusion.'" I asked, "How does your porcelain face feel?" He carefully responded, "It's very delicate, like it could crack any minute, it is also very much like a mask. Today I put on face makeup, hair spray, eyes drops, my teeth are fake, they're all bonded. I don't want anyone to see I have flaws." When I asked how he felt about putting on the mask, he responded, "I'm angry that I have to do these things, to make myself beautiful, it's a mask and I want to break it. It's making up for my lack of success as an individual, my not being more physically developed, and my not being emotionally developed. That takes really hard work, not makeup."

Soon after, James spoke with his lover about his not being happy in their relationship, but this time he also expressed his feeling that this was in part because he was not happy with himself and the way he was leading his life. Though James initially minimized and underreported his use of alcohol and drugs, he had become more aware of the dangerous situations he was courting, especially when he drank alcohol and did drugs—cocaine, ecstasy, and poppers—with friends. He attended AA and NA, albeit grudgingly, because his denial concerning his substance abuse and his high risk for HIV infection was gradually breaking down.

He was frightened of his capacity to delude himself about how much he was at risk for contracting HIV. On one occasion, he had unprotected sex with a friend when the friend reassured him that they had nothing to worry about because he had recently tested negative. When he later discussed this experience with me, he felt confused and dismayed by his denial. James scheduled himself for an HIV test approximately 14 months after we had started working together. His test returned negative once again, though it was clearer to him that he was playing Russian roulette with his life.

We discussed the many ways in which he sought to disown his sense of purposefulness while getting others to tell him what to do, then rebelling against their control, most often in a self-destructive manner. For example, he described going out to dinner with a female friend who insisted that he should not have more than one glass of wine. In the moment, he acquiesced, behaving like a cute little boy who expected to be scolded, as if he appreciated not only her concern, but also her stern control over him. After dinner, however, they went their separate ways, and he was gradually aware of how resentful he felt about her control. Feeling infantilized and humiliated, he walked to a nearby bar, had several drinks in angry determination, and spent the evening with a young man he met there. They had reportedly used condoms during intercourse.

At times during our discussion of how James felt about the possibility of becoming infected with HIV, he would speak of God. At times he felt God was his protector and would keep him from harm through infection. Within this protective fantasy he also experienced our work, and his sense that I cared about him, as a protective shield from becoming infected. For example, during one session in which he was expressing his belief that I cared about him and that this helped him value himself and his life, he communicated the following: " With you, I feel that I am wanted. I feel that God loves me too much and wouldn't give it [HIV] to me, although almost everyone around me has gotten it. I know I have to protect myself, but still, I have this feeling of being protected because many others have turned positive and I haven't."

James also maintained the opposite view, of a God who objected to his sexual orientation and lifestyle, and who would sooner or later punish him. From this perspective, James expressed the fantasy that HIV represents a divine punishment for homosexuality as sinful, particularly within his own Catholic background. I recommended that he read up on this subject, letting him know that I had recently found a book by John Boswell (1980) about Christianity and homosexuality quite thorough and interesting. He asked if he could borrow the book, and I agreed, after a discussion of what it meant for him to do so. As a personal exchange, the book represented my lending him support and acceptance of his need to communicate about the particular struggles he faced in being Catholic and gay. Boswell's book traces the changing views of homosexuality over time within the Catholic church. Learning that his struggles have a social history enabled James to gain a broader perspective from which to examine his own feelings about these issues, and this underscored his ties to others with similar concerns.

As James became more aware and interested in learning to identify and express his own wishes and aspirations, as well as his underlying desire for domination and control of others, he became more assertive in a wide variety of circumstances. After several months of looking for a better job, he was hired in a more challenging and higher paying position. James also became more assertive about his being gay. He joined a gay men's basketball team in which he initially felt quite unsure of his ability, but gradually came to feel he was an integral part of the team. He also joined a gay men's therapy group, but dropped out after several months, feeling the other members were too confronting and judgmental of his lifestyle. He was more verbal about his differences with his family, his desire for their acceptance of his sexual orientation, and was not as tolerant of abuse from others. In his relationship with his lover, he expressed greater distress about being the target of hostility, and was deriving less pleasure from their sadomasochistic interactions.

I was on vacation when I received a message from James on my answering machine; his most recent test results indicated he had become HIV-positive and had also contracted hepatitis B. Deeply pained by the weight and severity of this news, I returned his call after a brief period of reflection. We shared deep feelings of grief, recognizing that this tragic turn in his life had taken place just as he was beginning to gain a greater sense of self and, thereby, a greater sense of command over his destiny.

James and I met a few days after our phone contact. Initially James fluctuated between states of shock and bouts of intense worrying and depression. I, in turn, struggled privately with feelings of grief and helplessness, but I counterbalanced these feelings with the hope of helping James maximize his chances of improving his emotional and physical health. Despite powerful shifts in mood, his determination to find out everything he could about the nature of the virus remained consistent. I was struck by the command and immediacy with which he had taken over the situation; he had secured treatment with an HIV specialist and had found a second physician to treat his hepatitis. Furthermore, he had been reading updates on medical treatments, and was also discussing a number of nonmedical approaches with friends who had sought alternative treatments. Within the first month of turning positive, he received massage therapy, acupuncture for stimulation of immune functioning, and was looking into vitamin C drips, gamma globulin intravenous treatment, and relevant nutritional information. During this turbulent period, James was very proud to have been able to hold on to his full-time job. He had taken several weeks off to recover from his hepatitis infection, and returned to work as soon as he was medically cleared.

James's initial shock gave way to increased feelings of depression. Although his ability to get up-to-date medical information and treatment helped alleviate his anxiety, his attention then shifted toward the broader emotional impact of his seroconversion. James struggled with feelings of self-recrimination. Whereas he felt the work he was doing in his analysis was helping him, he was painfully aware that it was too late to guard his life against this terrifying turn. His profound grief stretched from his present feelings of loss to an earlier, more innocent, and barely awakened consciousness about his own mortality. Recalling his previous fantasy about the lion and the zebra, he poignantly expressed his feeling that it was all to have been a "playing out" of the fantasy of being devoured, desired perhaps to the point of annihilation. He had previously wondered if perhaps through this total surrender and union he would be loved. He was now more acutely aware of not yet having established a lasting sense of closeness to a loving partner, and of not having achieved a feeling of belonging in the world.

I struggled with feeling that I should have been able to prevent this situation from occurring. As his therapist, I thought I could have done so by being more adamant or forceful in the manner in which I communicated my objection to high-risk behaviors, including his substance abuse. I had previously consulted with a number of colleagues about this issue. One senior clinician said that if a patient of his continued to take such risks in his sexual behavior, he would flatly tell the patient to desist or else discontinue their work together. I felt this would have resulted in full reenactment, turning the therapist into the punitive and controlling older brother or parental figure, which would limit the opportunity for dialogue and exploration.

James was gradually able to express some of his anger toward me about his turning positive. He voiced my own fear that perhaps he wouldn't have turned positive had I been more forceful and dominant toward him in the treatment. He expressed his craving for a more authoritarian approach from me, feeling that this would have helped protect him from his impulsivity and reckless self-abandon. I withstood his immediate anger and resentment, while I continued to work through my own feelings and thoughts about my approach to our work. At other times, James asserted that were I to have become more directive, he would have either terminated the treatment earlier or would have gone on a binge of sexual exploits to let me know just who was to be in charge.

James let his mother know of his HIV status early on, and tested the waters for informing his father. His mother supported his reticence to tell his father, fearing that this news would plunge his father into a deep depression. James was also reluctant to directly acknowledge his homosexuality with his father. In part, he feared that his being HIV-positive would underscore his father's view of his homosexuality as something sinful and malignant. He did inform his father of his having hepatitis B, and in this manner he opened the door for them to interact around his being ill. His mother accompanied him to medical appointments and his father was also quite supportive. At times, however, his mother lashed out at James, blaming him for his illness and the emotional turmoil he brought her. After a particularly heated argument with his mother, she had blurted out, "Everything that goes wrong in this house is your fault!" In our session, James stated, "I just don't want anyone in my life who's that angry. It's really toxic. It reminds me of the abusive way I treated myself. No matter how painful it was to walk away from her, I got up and left her. I felt I had to break the cycle. Later I thought, 'God, I hope you can forgive me for leaving her behind.'"

Prior to his seroconversion, James had turned to prayer for consolation and hope. Following his seroconversion, the frequency of his praying and his feelings about his relationship to God were intensified. At times, he felt his turning positive represented a punishment from God for his periods of self-indulgence and his homosexuality. However, he was also able to turn to God as a source of soothing protection. Although at times he regarded his seroconversion as a death sentence, he also perceived it as a challenge to establish a healthier, more productive and fulfilling life: "I believe that God closes some doors and opens others," he said, expressing that perhaps he would find greater strength to pursue his interests and establish a loving and lasting relationship, now that he felt more acutely aware of the value of his life and the passing of time.

As James continued to plummet into depressive feelings, he also seemed to be acknowledging truths that were difficult to confront. Each confrontation toward asserting himself delineated the painful boundary between himself and others. For example, James's HIV status represented a new barrier between us: "I'm positive and you are not. I can't bring you into my world, and you can't take me out of mine into yours." His seroconversion further propelled him to take a more assertive and unmasking role in his relationships: "I want to be the tough guy. . . . For all this suffering, what I'm gaining is a really deep sense of self."

The intensification of James's depressive feelings, which included periodic difficulty falling asleep, warranted our discussion of a psychopharmacological consultation. We agreed that he would see a psychiatrist who was familiar with treating depression in patients who are HIV-positive, but the psychiatrist felt James's symptoms did not warrant medication at this time. However, he also expressed concern for James's tendency toward substance abuse, correctly forewarning that this would increase as he recovered from his hepatitis and felt better.

As James recovered from hepatitis, he started dating a man whom he described as gentle, supportive, and complimentary, but he also let this man know that he was not emotionally ready for a new relationship. The intensity of his relationship with Scott had greatly diminished. Throughout this time, we continued to speak of the importance of safer sex practices and of abstinence from alcohol and drugs. In addition to his concern about not passing the virus on to others, we discussed the importance of keeping his viral load as low as possible, to minimize the possibility of infection with multiple strains of the virus, as well as to limit infection with other sexually transmitted diseases. With my encouragement, James entered a Body Positive 12-week support group. He found the group helpful in enabling him to address his immediate experience and to share with others who were dealing with similar circumstances.

Nearing the end of our second year of treatment, James announced, "I wanted to tell you I'm not going to see you anymore, yet I'm happy to see you. Either way I'm going to die, I want to get rid of this virus. You tell me to be truthful and I feel I hate everyone, I don't even like the music I used to listen to anymore. Yet, I looked in the mirror the other day and felt I really liked myself, as if for the first time." A couple of months later, James again expressed feelings of anger toward me, but more pointedly addressed his frustration about the irreversibility of his HIV status, especially as he experienced this in my presence. The magical soothing he had been able to achieve by fantasizing that our work would protect him was shattered. "You can't make me negative!" he voiced with resentment. In the meantime, he continued to educate himself on the nature of HIV. He borrowed a book of mine on cell biology, in order to study the important aspects of the virus which may be implicated in a future cure.

James wanted to become more independent from me, without fully losing contact with me. The books he borrowed were valuable to him for the knowledge they imparted regarding the topics we were discussing in treatment, yet they also seemed to serve as transitional objects, particularly during a time when he was considering taking steps toward separation from me. With my agreement and support, he decided to reduce our sessions to twice a week, and a year later, to once a week. During this time he also entered brief treatment with a gay psychologist who specialized in working with men in abusive relationships. James was initially concerned (and was secretly hoping) that my feelings would be hurt, that I would be narcissistically wounded about my abilities as a therapist, as well as being jealous of his spending less time with me. His ability to voice these concerns reduced his fears. He also reluctantly acknowledged that his wish to push me away was an expression of his anger for my not having prevented his turning positive. He emphasized, however, that he felt proud of his having completed two years of treatment on a three times a week basis; we agreed that it was important not to lose sight of this accomplishment and of the gains he had made thus far in his therapy.

Near the end of our second year of treatment, James also became concerned with trying to recapture and restore an original sense of self. For example, he was having fantasies about returning to the plastic surgeon who had performed cosmetic surgery on his nose years before, and to see if it could be made the same shape it had been prior to the surgery. This may have been motivated partly by his desire to revert to his self prior to HIV infection. During this period he reported several dreams in which he was meeting with his high school peers as an adult, feeling confident about himself. He felt he was reclaiming his feeling of popularity and belonging, feelings he had experienced with his peers during grammar school, but which were submerged following repeated experiences of ostracism during high school. He was less comfortable with "wearing a mask," with being seductive and acquiescent, and he summoned the courage to be more frank with others about his likes and dislikes.

James joined a long-term, dynamically oriented support group for HIV-positive gay men during the fourth year of our working together. He continued to struggle with periodic abuse of alcohol and cocaine, for which he sporadically attended 12-step meetings. Group therapy provided him with a forum within which to contrast his views with those of peers about a wide range of topics, ranging from his approach to treatment of his HIV to considerations about the impact of his HIV status on establishing new friendships and personal relationships. James and I terminated after four and a half years of treatment, maintaining an open door to our working together in the future, should he deem this helpful. I took pleasure in the ways that he was coming to life, including his increased ability to make choices with greater autonomy and capacity for self-reflection; yet I also felt steeped in sadness when I considered the likelihood that his life would be foreshortened.

James emerged from our work better able to integrate the fragmented and fragile selves manifested through his defensive use of masks. Though our work did not prevent his becoming HIV-positive, James stands to live out the balance of his life with a greater sense of appreciation and care for himself and others. James helped me become more aware of the ways in which I too benefit from wearing masks, at times as camouflage and at times as an attempt to try on new ways of being. As therapists, our ability both to accept the masks that our patients try on and to embrace the various selves that lie behind them is crucial to facilitate their release from their particular form of bondage.

References

Benjamin, J. (1988), *The Bonds of Love.* New York: Pantheon Books.

Boswell, J. (1980), *Christianity, Social Tolerance, and Homosexuality.* Chicago, IL: University of Chicago Press.

Browning, F. (1994), *The Culture of Desire.* New York: First Vintage Books.

11 A Heterosexual Male Therapist's Journey of Self-Discovery

Wearing a "Straight"jacket in a Gay Men's Bereavement Group

John V. O'Leary

Since the onset of AIDS, 343,000 Americans, six times the number of soldiers killed in Vietnam, have died of it. Just as in that war, most of these men died when their lives were just getting started, "cut down in their prime" as the saying goes. This chapter is partly about those they left behind, their families, their lovers and their friends. It is about wounds that refuse to heal, grief that cannot be assuaged. I do not emphasize technical strategies, curative factors, or even personal breakthroughs, of which there were some. I deal mostly with countertransference issues. I describe a journey of self-discovery, one with which some of my readers can identify. I believe there is much that we can learn from our encounters with traumatized people (Schaffner, 1994); those immediately affected by the AIDS crisis are no exception.

The group I discuss started in October 1994 as part of the HIV Clinical Service under the directorship of Dr. Mark Blechner. The HIV Clinical Service is an outreach program at the William Alanson White Institute in New York City. The group meets in my office once a week for an hour and a half and has an open-door policy for new members. The duration of the group is intended to be long term.

The group comprises gay men in their 30s and 40s who have suffered profound personal losses. These men are HIV-negative, that is, from an HIV perspective they are all counted among the "well." Most are college educated; all are white. Three of the men had extensive individual therapy before joining the group. Indeed, some were referred by their individual therapists.

The extent of the members' losses is difficult to convey. One man described losing his lover of seven years, as well as each of the six friends who had sat with him through that last vigil. My patient is a lone survivor. While this is the most dramatic case of multiple loss, his story resonates for all the members of the group and is a stark illustration of how their experiences go beyond ordinary grieving. Whereas loss is often a singular, albeit tragic, event in someone's life, these men face chronic loss, which has become an integral problem for the community to which they belong.

Despite the devastation of these losses, they are not the only source of my clients' grief. Other significant losses have been part of the social matrix of the bereaved gay man. First, gay men are losing a lifestyle that many grew up taking for granted. This includes homosexual courtship, mating, and lovemaking rituals. The term "safe sex" hardly conveys what has changed in homosexual society. Each new social encounter now raises many questions: Is this person HIV-positive? Was he ever tested? Will he tell me the truth? Will he practice safe sex? Is his understanding of safe sex the same as mine? What if I fall in love and he comes down with AIDS? Should I even bother getting involved when there is so much to worry about? Several of the men in my group have answered this last question with a resounding "no." They are extremely fearful, not just of contracting AIDS, but of putting themselves back on the path of worry. This is an especially pernicious loss because it impedes what is necessary for the natural mourning process, a reconnection with one's social network.

Another form of loss is the fall in status from a marginally accepted group to an even lower one. Many gay men see themselves as modern-day equivalents of carriers of the "black plague." Some grew up in a time when there seemed to be progress in gaining acceptance by the dominant, straight society. Gay rights legislation had passed in some states. Gay groups were active on most campuses. Many gay men had attained a post-"Stonewall" kind of pride. The advent of AIDS brought a new stigma. Now "coming out" is even more fraught with difficulty. Some gay men announce to their parents, in a macabre form of "double jeopardy," that they are both gay and HIV-positive.

Facing the additional loss of efficacy on the job, all members of my group have reported career setbacks. They have had to take time off, and their supervisors frown on these sudden, unexplained absences as well as on what the employees themselves recognize as uninspired performances. Sometimes these absences have occurred because of the deteriorating health condition of their lovers, and sometimes because of their own depleted coping resources. Normally, a grieving employee can explain what is going on and will be given considerable latitude. Many gay men fear making these disclosures, with good reason. This secrecy, however, often results in the growing exasperation of their employers. Finally, these employees may find themselves bypassed for promotions, given smaller bonuses, subject to disciplinary action, or, in some cases, terminated.

There is a fourth loss I see, although this phenomenon is not usually described in terms of loss. Normally, when a person has undergone many traumas he feels a right to his sadness, anger, despair, or even detachment. The men in my group, particularly in early sessions, were deeply ashamed of these feelings—especially because of their HIV-negative status. After all, they were not sick. What right did they have to feel sorry for themselves? They had been spared. "Survivor guilt" takes the form of accusing oneself of being more justly deserving of AIDS than the loved one, given one's own "promiscuous" behavior. This attitude has been reinforced over the several years when they were primary caregivers. The PWA (person with AIDS) was the center of everyone's attention. The partners (i.e., my patients) were seen by others and saw themselves as members of the "worried well," and thus more fortunate.[1]

There are other losses, such as the loss of the ceremonial rituals that occur when someone has died and that help provide closure for the survivors. Some of these men had their caretaking roles powerfully and abruptly usurped in the final days by the lover's family of origin. Family members may displace the lover in planning funeral proceedings or memorial services. Even when the parents believe that the surviving

1. This term, the "worried well," has taken on a few different meanings since the start of the HIV epidemic. At its earliest use, the term referred to those whose test results were negative, yet who still believed themselves to be positive. It also referred to those who always engaged in "safe sex," yet believed they would test positive. Another, more current meaning is more pejorative; it refers to those who seek out treatment for ailments that are trivial compared to the afflictions of those who are truly suffering.

lover is HIV-negative, they may associate him with a lifestyle that killed their child. This practice of exclusion from funeral plans is one source of the powerful rage toward straight society that I have heard expressed in the group.

I imagine by this time you see where I am going. The grief these men endure is insidious, ironically self-perpetuating, and complex. To a large extent it touches all gay men, regardless of their bereavement status.

It is important, I believe, to describe some of the lessons and surprises afforded me by my work with this group. As a member of the dominant culture, like other straight therapists (no matter their best intentions), I can fall prey to subtle prejudices, fears, and unrecognized homophobia (a term I prefer is "heterosexism"). In some instances, this attitude is built into the analytic models available to therapists and the therapeutic conventions that spring from recent pressures to be cost effective.

It is currently a fashionable idea in the United States that bereavement therapy works best on a short-term basis. Bereavement groups usually meet weekly for anywhere from 8 to 12 weeks. This model has many advocates (Piper, McCallum, and Azim, 1992; Sifneos, 1979) and includes many training programs, some within the homosexual community. Needless to say, this format is cost effective and is often presented in professional meetings as appealing to managed care companies. While this model is problematic for grieving under any circumstances (Yalom and Vinogradov, 1988), it is particularly ill-suited for gay clients. Mourning a loss to AIDS does not have the circumscribed quality seen in mainstream culture. Multiple and ongoing losses are now the rule rather than the exception in gay culture. To insist on a short-term group for gay mourners is to imply that continued grieving is pathological, particularly when it goes on well past the prescribed 12 weeks. What is most important, this time limit operates in unconscious collusion with survivor guilt and the entrenched belief of HIV-negative men that intensive treatment should be reserved for the truly sick, that is, for those who are HIV-positive.

A second example pertains to the neutrality and anonymity of the analytic group leader. When I started this group, I was somewhat uncomfortable as a straight man leading a group of exclusively gay men, but I convinced myself that it ought not matter. My neutrality and anonymity prevented me from discussing my personal life. I certainly intended to be neutral (in Bion's [1970] sense of "having no memory nor desire") and to deal with issues as they came up. Also, I tried to convince myself that this group was primarily about grief, and I *did* know something about that.

I recognized an overt clue, however, that I was far less secure in these beliefs than I had admitted to myself. I wanted very much to find a gay cotherapist who had "come out," a colleague who could be clear to the group about his identity. When the cotherapist idea fell through, my anxiety—I won't say it went through the roof—certainly approached the ceiling. Nevertheless, when the group began to meet, I was the solo therapist. I was very relieved that no one in those early days asked me about my sexual orientation. I realized much later that the group members didn't ask me about it because they generally presumed I was gay. Who else would run a group exclusively for gay men? Had the group been composed of gay and straight people, they could reasonably have presumed I was straight. Also, inasmuch as training institutes generally have excluded gay candidates, if an analyst is operating in mainstream psychoanalysis, chances are that he is straight. What is important is that these beliefs reflect social reality and are not transference distortions.

Over time I found that my anonymity became a serious obstacle to my natural responsiveness. I didn't want to say anything that would give away my sexual identification, but so many things that people talked about brought it up. Parallels and metaphors from my straight life were not working, and I began to feel like an outsider, or, even worse, an interloper. At times I pretended to understand jargon that I didn't. At the same time, I was developing a genuine admiration for these men. They seemed heroic to me. I wondered if I could do what they had done when the chips were down, staying with people through endless crises. Would I have the heart for that?

This may seem naive to many because it came so late in the process, but after weeks of this, I suddenly realized that I was reliving, in abbreviated form, what for gay men was a constant experience in their relationship to the heterosexual world. Like them, I wondered if I was "passing." I was twisting myself into a pretzel to make sure I was. Was I beginning to feel a need to "come out" as straight? At the time, it seemed unthinkable! I remember impassioned discussions about having good gay role models. I had images of everyone in the group quitting if I revealed myself as heterosexual.

Around this time, I sought supervision. As you might guess, this wasn't easy. I couldn't find a single male therapist in the same situation I was in. There were quite a few women who were running groups for HIV-positive gay men, but by and large, their sexual orientations were not in question (or at least, I didn't think so). Fortunately, I did find excellent supervision through the auspices of the Eastern Group Psychotherapy Society (EGPS). The main outcome of that was to stop pretending to know things I didn't. If the group members gathered that I was straight from my uninformed questions, so be it. I would free myself from my straight jacket.

As most of us know, however, life travels faster than supervision, and two sessions later, one of the newer members popped the question.

"Dr. O'Leary, are you straight or gay?" Unfortunately, he did not do this during a formal session, but during a small postsession Christmas party that we decided to have—when none of my analytic props were available. (I just wasn't going to ask at a party, "What does that bring up for you?") We were all still seated in a circle, lest you think I had some privacy in answering his question. There was nothing for me to do but answer honestly and, I might add, with great relief. It did help to share with them the painful struggle of the previous months, and how it had taught me something about what they were going through. To my genuine surprise and pleasure, no one quit the group.

Something did change after that session. Members brought in much more concrete material about their sexual lives or their yearnings for it. I began to hear about one-night stands, sex club activity, and masturbation fantasies. There also seemed to be a lot more humor in the group. They kidded with me about the decor of my office and how only a straight man could tolerate so many aesthetic incongruities. Not only was I freed from the weight of analytic neutrality, but the group seemed to loosen up with their knowledge as well. Everything felt more real.

I started this discussion about revealing my sexual identity with the observation that parallels and metaphors from my straight life were not working for me in the group. I would like to elaborate on that statement. I will say at the outset that I am unsure how much of this lack of congruency can be attributed to my upbringing in mainstream homophobic society and how much was the result of psychoanalytic conventions. I have come to believe that the two mutually reinforced each other. At any rate, I shall mention some serious biases that I brought to this group.

The most pervasive I have noticed are, first, the belief that sexual identity is always a learned or acquired phenomenon. I originally pictured male homosexuality as a choice facilitated by family constellations (e.g., a rejecting father, an intrusive, controlling mother). Second, I held the attitude that monogamous and exclusive relationships are necessarily the preferred mode of being, a sort of psychological "best fit," for both straight and gay societies. Finally, I believed that the personal and the political are separate modes of experience. Most of what is important about one's life is lived outside of the domain of politics—or so I believed.

Sexual Identity: Learned versus Innate

Consider the first issue, that of sexual identity formation. Some may disagree, but I believe that most psychoanalytic therapists have left the narrow corridor of "homosexuality equals psychopathology." Even classical analysts are loath to defend this aspect of their history, although some still do, as witness Socarides and Volkan (1995). Nonetheless, I propose there is a reassessment, no mere attempt at political correctness, but a genuine effort to rid our discipline of intellectually indefensible positions. Unfortunately, what goes out the front door sometimes reappears at the back, where we meet again the residue of a developmental theory that explains sexual object choice in terms of oedipal theory, the failure to identify with the father.

What makes this theory so hard to dispel is that its premises are often borne out by therapists' work with gay patients. All of the men in my group have reported difficulties with their fathers. Some fathers appear downright sadistic in the accounts given by their sons. I have heard many stories of ill-tempered fathers who seemed to enjoy humiliating their children in front of the entire family. One father, for example, banged his son's head down onto the dining table on a regular basis, simply to illustrate his control over the household. Other fathers seem detached or narcissistically preoccupied.

From these disclosures, too, I learned of an experience common to many group members. They reported the powerful "sense of being different" that dates from their earliest memories. They were different from their siblings, different from their playmates. Many felt alienated from the rough-and-tumble of boys' games and could not identify with stereotypical male images. Some describe being drawn instead to play with little girls. Few would acknowledge these feelings to their parents; some tried and even succeeded at mastery over sports. These men believed that their fathers would never be able to accept them for who they were. It was as if their fathers recognized them through the facade and hated them for it.

Hearing it cast this way, I started reexamining the lens through which I viewed sexual identity development. If you put homosexuality first, as a genetic given, and poor fathering second, just as compelling a case can be made for homosexuality causing troubled parenting. It made sense to me that in our homophobic society, some men would view an effeminate son (a "sissy") as the worst thing that could happen. But perhaps these sons were unable to receive whatever emotional cues their fathers offered. Such fathers, detecting this lack of reciprocity, would emotionally detach themselves, not feeling connected in the culturally prescribed way. The more disturbed the father, or the more he was attached to "machismo," the more these dissonances would spark overt cruelty. While I now know this sequence of experience has been keenly described by a few in the analytic literature, such as Isay, I was hearing, for the first time, personal accounts that supported this theory.

Some men described their mothers' efforts to protect them from their fathers. Is this the "overprotective mother" described in the earlier analytic literature? Some men felt their mothers were trying to assume the roles of both mother and father to them. Is this the "intrusive mother" we so often hear about? For other men, however, their mothers were not protective. These men felt adrift from both parents, and they seemed to have the most trouble in the group. One man, who had run away from home and been on his own for several years, has left the group, suddenly and without warning, for weeks at a time. The group finds him difficult to get to know. He is the most isolated member of the group.

I am less sure today about this genetic hypothesis; I have since read many convincing arguments against this "essentialist" position. For example, some feminist postmodernist writers (Dimen, 1991; Harris, 1991; Burch, 1993) reject the idea of a unified or coherent gender identity. Instead, these thinkers have incorporated notions of fluidity and multiplicity in their understandings of gender experience. Nonetheless, what I am highlighting here is the recognition of the rigidity of my earlier views.

Monogamy: Acting Out versus Open Relationships

I move now to the second bias I brought to the group: the overvaluation of monogamy. I remember the first time Adam, a group member, spoke of reconnecting with an old sexual partner. It was his first foray into the sexual arena after years of abstinence. My relief and hope for him were brought up short when I learned that the intended liaison was with Dale, a man who was still living with his lover of five years. Adam expressed some guilt about this, but he quickly moved on to other aspects of their relationship. I anticipated that the group would challenge Adam on the wisdom of this choice, given the number of available, unattached men. Instead, they simply asked about the nature of the arrangement. Adam said that Dale would take a weekend off every couple of months and fly to another city. Dale had made it clear that questions were not welcome from Dale's lover about these sojourns. Someone joked that maybe "while the cat was away the mouse would play."

Since I also run a group for heterosexuals, I was struck by what seemed to be a cavalier attitude about this matter. My other group would have presented a powerful challenge to the group member about "acting out" and "avoidance of intimacy," questioning how and why he would begin a relationship that could go nowhere. They would not have been reassured by the rules of the "arrangement." Indeed, they would also have questioned the group member about why he would want someone so unwilling to make a commitment.

Straight society puts a psychological premium on coupling and monogamy. This attitude is reflected in the prevailing analytic attitude. Breaks from monogamy are seen as "acting out" or "flights from intimacy." It seemed to me that the men in my bereavement group allowed for much greater flexibility on these issues. I came to see that there is a spectrum of possible relationships in gay culture that reflects individual style and how men contract with their partners. This may come out of some aspects of male-to-male bonding that we do not understand yet. For example, one couple had the rule that each partner could sleep with anyone else he wanted, but only as a "one-night stand." I am not suggesting there is no jealousy in such situations. On the contrary, some of these "arrangements" set the stage for intense conflict. The jealousy does seem better tolerated, however, and less likely to result in the breakup of the relationship.

Political and Personal: Continuous or Separate Realities?

The final issue pertains to my beliefs about the personal versus the political. I remember one session in November that I found particularly unsettling. The men were talking about loneliness. Each was describing in the most vivid terms how alone he felt in the world. Some felt old and used up, believing that the "good times" had passed them by. Others felt that death hung over them like a black cloud and no one could stand to be around them. Each account seemed to touch off emotions in the other members. I don't think any of us were dry-eyed during this session.

About two-thirds into the session, one of the men brought up the topic of the 1994 political elections. I immediately considered the topic inappropriate, given the intense feeling of the group at that moment. All that kept me from intervening was my knowledge of the person who had brought it up. Usually he is not emotionally tuned out. Nonetheless, I wondered what, in this very intimate engagement, he was running away from.

To my surprise, the group took up this political question with considerable intensity. They were extremely angered and saddened by the elections, which had brought a conservative (translate, "reactionary," "antigay") majority into the House of Representatives and the Senate.

They saw the results as devastating on a local level, bearing extremely bad tidings for them. I had also been disappointed by the results, but on a more strictly intellectual level. I didn't really understand the group's concern. As I sat in bewilderment, the men in the group tied this experience in with their intense feelings of loneliness. They did not hear the election topic as differentiated from their previous sentiments. The elections stood as further proof that no one cared for them. It underscored their loneliness. The whole of American society seemed hostilely allied against them. They could expect little or nothing from outsiders. For the next five minutes, I don't think I heard anything that was said. I was searching desperately for some kind of anchor to bring me back into the discussion. Fortunately, the session came to an end. I had a week to process what had happened.

I'm still not sure what to make of this dysfunction or failure in empathy, if indeed it was a failure, but I have some thoughts about it. I believe our natural mind-set as psychotherapists is to highlight and accentuate what is most personal and idiosyncratic. We search for family enactments in our patients as well as in ourselves. Although many of our teachers, such as Harry Stack Sullivan and Erich Fromm, stressed the powerful forces that impinge from the outside, we tend to award little credibility to them in any given therapy hour. It is easier to maintain this posture when the swing of political forces makes little difference to us personally. Republican or Democrat, we lead our lives pretty much as usual. Only issues of national health insurance seemed to intensify the political drama that year for psychotherapists. I think most members of the mainstream feel this same way about political issues. There is the personal, and then there is the political. The former is serious and compelling. The latter can be fascinating, infuriating, occasionally inspiring, but ultimately, removed from daily life. The injunction not to discuss baseball or politics rests on this premise.

Politics and personal life are of one piece. To oppressed minorities, the course of political developments is a symbolic expression of how we feel about them personally. I can better appreciate this as a result of my experience with this group.

To sum up, I have worked toward a more respectful stance with my gay clients, one that recognizes profound differences in cultural experience. We cannot do psychoanalytic work effectively if we are bound by some of the cultural biases I have discussed. We must make adaptations in analytic technique in light of these difficulties.

In the individual psychoanalytic literature I have found the most viable model in the writings of Racker (1968), Sandler (1976), Hoffman (1983), Blechner (1992), Levenson (1991), Hirsch (1995), and a few others. Sometimes labeled "radical countertransference," this theory posits that the analyst is deeply entwined with the patient's unconscious from the outset. The analyst remains alert to unconscious collusion with the patient who frequently carries negative, stereotypical self-images.

I have provided just a few examples of such collusions. My readiness to see pathology in the family as the primary cause of homosexual identity formation unconsciously supported the group members' belief that their families of origin had done them immeasurable harm. In another instance, many of these men saw themselves as incapable of forming new, stable, and loving relationships. I was unconsciously prepared to reinforce that cynical belief by holding them to a rigid heterosexual standard.

What rescued me from some of these follies was a willingness to admit I was in uncharted territory. I did not trust my footing and could take little for granted. I had no cotherapist, the standard grief models seemed hopelessly inadequate, and neutrality and anonymity had not worked. The men in this group were constantly telling me important things about themselves. Occasionally I dropped my preconceptions and just listened and learned.

References

Bion, W. R. (1970), *Attention and Interpretation.* London: Heinemann.

Blechner, M. J. (1992), Working in the countertransference. *Psychoanal. Dial.,* 2:161–179.

Burch, B. (1993), Gender identity, lesbianism, and potential space. *Psychoanal. Psychol.,* 10:359–375.

Dimen, M. (1991), Deconstructing difference: Gender splitting and transitional space. *Psychoanal. Dial.,* 1:335–352.

Harris, A. (1991), Gender as contradiction. *Psychoanal. Dial.,* 1:197–224.

Hirsch, I. (1995), Therapeutic uses of countertransference. In: *Handbook of Interpersonal Psychoanalysis,* ed. M. Lionells, J. Fiscalini, C. Mann & D. Stern. Hillsdale, NJ: The Analytic Press, pp. 643–660.

Hoffman, I. Z. (1983), The patient as interpreter of the analyst's experience. *Contemp. Psychoanal.,* 19:389–422.

Isay, R. A. (1990), *Being Homosexual.* New York: Avon Books.

Levenson, E. (1991), *The Purloined Self.* New York: Contemporary Psychoanalysis Books.

Piper, W. E., McCallum, M. & Azim, H. F. A. (1992), *Adaptation to Loss Through Short-Term Psychotherapy.* New York: Guilford.

Racker, H. (1968), *Transference and Countertransference.* New York: International Universities Press.

Sandler, J. (1976), Countertransference and role responsiveness. *Internat. Rev. Psycho-Anal.*, 3:43–47.

Schaffner, B. (1994), The crucial and difficult role of the psychotherapist in the treatment of the HIV-positive patient. *J. Amer. Acad. Psychoanal.*, 22:505–518.

Sifneos, P. E. (1979), *Short-Term Dynamic Psychotherapy Evaluation and Technique.* New York: Plenum.

Socarides, C. & Volkan, V. (1995), *The Homosexualities and the Therapeutic Process.* Madison, CT: International Universities Press.

Yalom, I. D. & Vinogradov, S. (1988), Bereavement groups: Techniques and themes. *Internat. J. Group Psychother.*, 38:419–446.

12 Dances with Men

The Impact of Multiple Losses in My Practice of Psychoanalytically Informed Psychotherapy

Susan Bodnar

It was close to the end of my day on the inpatient AIDS unit at Roosevelt Hospital. I was a postdoctoral fellow in consultation liaison psychology. I felt I had just moved to a different country. Even though the hospital unit wasn't another geographic destination, it was a unique symbolic culture. This day, like most others, I had struggled to understand and to communicate in a version of my native language that contained inferences and references that were foreign to me. Death hovered in the air so palpably that it lingered on my clothes.

Mr. R, one of my first therapy patients, was confident that he had beaten yet another AIDS-related opportunistic infection. He was an energetic gay man about to return home. He often entertained staff and patients with his Martha and the Vandellas routine. He would don a black wig and croon a few tunes. Wry and wise, he interpreted the behavior of staff members like a Ouija board. If an aide left the room without looking at him, he interpreted, "Scared and tired." If his nurse administered medication too efficiently, he commented, "Your studied nonchalance is unbecoming. Look at me like you know me."

While he packed and readied himself for his discharge, we spoke about bicycling. He was a mountain bike enthusiast, and urged me to try it. "It's too bumpy," I said. "It ruins the view."

"That's just the point," he responded with a wink. "You've got to look between the bounces and enjoy what you can."

In one of those inexplicable doctor-patient reversals, I felt understood. Mr. R had no way of knowing that the man to whom I had been married for eight years had died from cancer one year before. I came to work in the medical psychology field because my experience with terminal illness generated new psychological questions. In addition, people in their early 30s dominated my professional and social world. My colleagues and friends weren't questioning life or making sense of death. Fearful of becoming a dour and depressive dinner companion, or an unusually intense psychologist, I sought companions who witnessed life between the bounces. The knowledge that life is finite had transported me to the poet's interior palace.

Entering the Field

I remembered Mr. R two years later when I pulled an index card from a stack of hundreds stamped with hospital data. "Mr. R, DOB 9/1/60," it said. Almost 66 percent of the people whose names appeared on those cards died within the year. Each name etched faces into my memory as clearly as the purple imprint on the white card. The cards symbolized people I knew and the lessons they passed on to me. Most of my patients were gay men of various backgrounds. Many of the doctors and staff with whom I worked and who supervised me were also gay men. It was a rare encounter with myself as a minority. Despite the commonality of human experience and the large social categories that united all people, distinct cultural differences existed between my life as a heterosexual woman and the lives of the men I came to know.

The impact of AIDS was only one of those differences. For me, AIDS had been something on the news that only gradually made its way into my everyday awareness. The staff on the inpatient unit had coped with it as a reality from the epidemic's incipience. Many of the physicians had organized the first responses to the AIDS crisis and had lost people they loved to the disease's wrenching grip. Most still struggled for legitimacy in a society that didn't quite know what to do with its homosexual and lesbian members. Here on the AIDS unit, those ordinarily stigmatized individuals, patients and physicians alike, were my teachers, my guides, my mentors, and my rabbis.

My colleagues understood life from the perspective of death. The doctors, nurses, lovers, friends, families, and spouses had been steeped in one of the worst medical crises in modern history. They invented a language to express death and what it feels like to die with someone. That language reinvented hierarchical relationships as something more collaborative. The ordinary boundaries between professional and personal life were unusually permeable.

My first week on the unit was exhausting—the pace frantic, the nurses loud and funny, and the medical doctors serious. Red lights blinked. Alarmed nurses exchanged glances. Hands waved, fingers pointed, and faces paled. Doctors wrote chart notes in mysterious code: squiggles, formulas, and abbreviated groupings of letters. Specialists rushed in and out of patient rooms. Large pieces of diagnostic machinery careened around corners. People yelled and people laughed. People cried. Yet an odd silence fell upon the nurses' station when I entered it. No one read my chart notes either.

My very first consultation was with a middle-aged man. He looked aghast when I strode into his room. I explained that his physician had sent me to speak with him. He seemed uncomfortable. I smiled pleasantly and proceeded to explain my purpose, earnestly. He winced. I gently explained that I knew it was hard to talk about complicated issues like illness, but perhaps we could begin by my asking a few questions.

"No, it's not that," he barked. "I'm urinating."

Sure enough, that was a portable latrine upon which he was perched. Thus began my crash course on boundaries.

Peter, a gregarious, stocky nurse with teddy bears pinned to his colorful clothing, rescued me later that day. He put his arm around me and took me to the back room. He called me "sweetie." What did sweetie mean? I wondered. Was it a term of endearment or one of disrespect?

"Sweetie," he said, "it happens to everybody. Get used to it, and keep your sense of humor." Then with a more menacing look he added, "You hetero girls—"

I thought, What is a hetero girl? Is it bad?

He continued, "Let me explain it to you this way, sweetie. We play by different rules here. Don't doctor-patient your patients, and lose the clipboard—yesterday." Thus began my system of carrying around discrete index cards on which I could keep important notes about my patients. I "lost" the clipboard, and a barrier behind which I could hide.

Peter became my friend and my advocate. He helped patients and doctors to feel relaxed about my presence. One day, Peter asked, "Why did you come here?" I didn't know what to say. My sense of professionalism urged me to describe an interest in mind-body interaction, especially the effect of psychological events on neurotransmitter activity. Instead, my gratitude for his help led me to tell the truth. I said, "I had a loss, and I didn't know what else to do." He asked for my story. I told him that at 29 years old, I had lost my husband of eight years.

The next day, the atmosphere changed. I noticed whispers and murmurs at the nurses' station: "She had a loss." Suddenly, I had friends. Later I understood that most of the people working on the unit had losses. Some had many. Newly aware of my widow's status, one of the physicians gave me a good looking over before spuriously commenting, "We play by the rules of life here, and you can't know what they are until you understand death, and what we deal with." He took me to see my first expired body. "This is death," he said. Then he whispered, "And this is life." He reached over and caressed his patient's brow. That night, Peter gave me a videotape. It was a show that had been broadcast on public TV about health-care workers who had HIV. Peter was one of the featured nurses.

My other important teacher was the unit psychiatrist, John. He taught me medicine and the underlying organic issues in treating people with AIDS. We spent long hours together going over charts and CAT scans and MRIs. He was open and direct as he instructed me in the writing of chart notes that could communicate with other medical staff. He encouraged me to suggest orders, like brain scans and blood tests. I accompanied him on his personal rounds. He consulted with me about difficult cases. Unlike other psychiatrists and physicians with whom I had previously worked, he treated me as an equal. We interacted as colleagues. He worked hard on himself. Being a gay man in a potentially prejudicial profession challenged him. Exposure to many intimate losses, including that of his father, caused him to rethink his priorities. He had time to train me, and he respected my abilities.

Early in my work, I developed a recurrent dream. I was on a dance floor, dressed in an outfit made of hospital scrubs. The room had hospital beds and IV stands around the edges. I was trying to dance. I knew the steps, but I couldn't seem to move. Every step was agitated and awkward. I had mastered the technique, but I couldn't perform it. I felt useless and paralyzed. Slowly the room filled with gay men who, one by one, became my dancing partners. They led me effortlessly around the room. All I had to do was hold on and follow. By the end of the dream, I was waltzing gracefully and flawlessly.

Saving Life

One afternoon, I was paged to a non-AIDS floor where a person with AIDS was staying due to overcrowding. I was asked to do a mental status consult to assess whether or not Mr. J's depression was affecting his competency to make medical decisions. The nursing staff was worried about Mr. J's suicidal thoughts. When I encountered Mr. J, he was breathing heavily. His speech was faint. What was audible sounded incoherent. Alarms went off in my head as I recalled John's careful teachings. This man wasn't suffering from a depression. He was dying. I went out to the nurses' station and gave orders for blood tests and vital signs. I spoke with such conviction and authority that my orders were immediately carried out before anyone realized I wasn't a medical doctor. Within minutes, it was discovered that Mr. J, a 23-year-old actor, was in renal failure. His depression was in actuality a mental decompensation due to kidney malfunction. He was transported to the Intensive Care Unit immediately. I paged John, so he could sign the orders, and he refused. "Let this one stay on the books," he said, leaving my signature on the orders. That night I went home in a thunderstorm. The clouds crashed. The lightning sliced into the sky. I lay awake, terrified by the grim responsibilities of my job. Mr. J didn't die. A week later, he went home to his lover. They sent me flowers.

This type of scenario repeated itself many times. Saving life was the medical unit's mission. This mission depended on the accurate transmission of information. People had to use authority with clarity and caution. I understood that knowledge and technique should never be arbitrarily asserted onto a person. When problems were solved by conforming the data to fit a solution, the results were disastrous. I learned that the detailed information of a circumstance often suggested the answers most applicable to the problem at hand. Every circumstance dictated its own response. The clinician's skill—and best use of authority—was in the ability to hear it. John had taught me to listen by listening to me.

Rather than acting on preconceived ideas, or on stimulating psychological theories, I looked, listened, and responded to the facts that faced me. I had once believed I could solve complicated problems by organizing the experience to conform to a meaning I understood. My work taught me to tolerate uncertainty until the authenticity of experience generated its own meaning. I could no longer diagnose a person medically or psychologically without first listening to a description of symptoms as attempts to communicate in the best way a lay person knows how. When Mr. J told his nurses, "I'm dying, I'm dying," he wasn't thinking of killing himself. He was really dying.

Saving life meant deferring psychotherapy to medical needs. Sessions had to be interrupted for important tests or treatments. Saving life also meant addressing depression. Mr. K's physician diagnosed him with an easily treatable infection. Morose and sad, Mr. K refused treatment. "It's over," he said. "There is no point."

His lover, L, argued with him. L insisted that there was much to live for. In addition to their love, their newly appointed home, and the dogs, Mr. K was writing an important book. He still refused treatment. Mentally competent, Mr. K had the right to his own choices. However, his sleeping patterns, eating habits, and mood indicated that he had a depression. During rounds, the residents and interns discussed a treatment course. They endlessly debated whether or not the depression was psychologically or metabolically induced. Mr. K's private doctor explained, "It doesn't matter. Treat the symptom."

I talked with Mr. K and L about medication for depression. Working in a couple's session, L begged Mr. K just to try it. He agreed. His depression resolved, and he accepted the treatment, which cleared up his infection. There were many instances when depression, dementia, and underlying metabolic problems created mood disorders that interfered with treatment. Sometimes saving a life meant an aggressive attack on the symptoms without completely understanding their roots. I developed a quick hand at transforming a person's psychopathology. The urgent threat to life shortened the time available for in-depth explorations. Medication and a direct use of analytic interpretations provided me with tools. I could build new interactions for my patients, which changed the way they related to others.

For example, Mr. B was 64 years old, very sick, and tired of living. He became mean and surly. He refused treatments, then mercilessly rang the bell at his bedside. He called hospital officials when his requests were ignored. He offered to buy his doctor an apartment on the top floor of his building, so that the doctor could be available upon demand. When I consulted on his case, Mr. B told me, "Get out." His personality drove people away. He became lonelier. Isolation increased his depression. This made him sicker, and he became angrier. It was a vicious behavioral cycle.

I didn't have the opportunity to know this man. I would have no chance to uncover hidden meanings, memories, or unconscious defenses. Yet, his life was in danger. It was my job to help responsibly, using my tools as an analytically oriented therapist. The second time I went to see him, he told me to get out again. This time I said, "If you hate yourself as much as you seem to, I can understand why you wouldn't want anybody to see you." I thought, "I hardly know this man. What right do I have to say this? He is going to explode."

He glared. I continued, "You are doing a great job at playing the irascible old man, and you are succeeding." He didn't tell me to get out. I decided to take a huge risk. Observing his age, I assumed that he might have conflicts about being gay. I offered an interpretation, "You are so conflicted about life as a gay man, you can't even begin to comprehend how to die as a gay man." Then, for no real reason, I suggested that he should ring his buzzer every half hour.

My interpretations about his behavior weren't necessarily right or wrong. They merely interested him, and their apparent intelligence appealed to him. He liked my strength. He cooperated. He rang his buzzer every half hour. I realized later that he was very conflicted about his dependency on others. The structured bell-ringing reassured him. The doctors and nurses weren't abandoning him. He really was afraid that he had pushed people away. The intervention gave him a new way of interacting with others, which elicited the care he needed. After he went home some weeks later, I discovered that he had followed up on some referral information. He was attending a support group.

Relationships

Mr. R, the bicycle enthusiast, was readmitted. This time he had lymphoma. He was skinnier and more subdued. He knew that most people don't survive AIDS-related lymphoma, but he wanted to try radiation. When I arrived for our appointment, I noticed that he had his day planner next to his bed. He was faithfully scheduling his day, as though it were an ordinary workweek. "It is my work," he snarled when I commented. He then explained that he really didn't want me to come and see him if I was going to insist on wearing that "dreary-faced mask." "Don't try to be an angel," he scolded. "Get off your high horse of do-good psychology and start becoming a human being." I happened to have worn my hair pulled back that day. He sneered, "You have a widow's peak."

I laughed, thinking he was even more perceptive than he realized. I knew that he was angry. I remembered how often my late husband bitterly cursed me through his short and devastating illness. The containment of his rage was my way of loving and supporting him. His anger was his desperate attempt to stay in control, to maintain his dignity, and to die with integrity. By doing psychotherapy with Mr. R, I was also loving this quirky young African-American man. My understanding of human intimacy broadened. I became comfortable with the love inherent in being someone's therapist.

Soon after, I met Mr. M. It was his fifth hospitalization. He and his lover had accounting jobs, one on Wall Street and one in Midtown. Mr. M came from a large Italian family. Although his homosexuality was not endorsed, he and his lover were loved and accepted by his family. Fruit flies endlessly hovered in his room because his family members perpetually delivered large, generous fruit baskets. During our work together he described a hobby. He and his lover made "Christmas balls," handmade tree ornaments. My curiosity prompted Mr. M's lover to bring some in to show me. They were outrageous—wild, colorful, and joyous. My enjoyment of these Christmas balls encouraged them both to share other parts of their lives with me. They told me about the early coming-out days in New York City. "It was wonderful," Mr. M said, "to go to clubs with other gay men and to dance in public. Who wanted to stop? It was so freeing, so fantastic, it was like an explosion of happiness." They described close friendships, intimacy, and community gatherings.

Their love of dance developed into a hobby, and soon, by day they were working in suits, and by night they were dancing in clubs with their pet boa constrictors.

"It's really great," Mr. M exclaimed, "a real release. I mean, it's just so wild."

I had never met anybody who had danced with a snake in a nightclub before. I wanted to know all about it. Somehow, they sensed my interest was not in jest. They also shared memories of the earlier, more spontaneous Halloween parades when Mr. M first appeared on a West Village balcony dressed as the Pope. In careful detail, Mr. M and his lover described what went into the construction of that costume: the double seams, the search for the right weight linen, the lining, the edging, and then the hat, of course, had to be absolutely perfect. For years they caricatured the Pope on the balcony to the delight of the dancing crowds below.

Recently, though, Mr. M had been too sick to play the Pope on Halloween. Things were different now, anyway. In previous years, the parade had been energized by a political current. The early flamboyance asserted the rights of gay people. Lately the parade had become too hedonistic, too "idolatrous." The spirit had changed.

A few days after telling me his story, Mr. M died unexpectedly. His lover sat quietly in his room until the sun rose. He walked alone down the long hospital corridor, the cardboard box filled with Christmas balls tucked under his arm.

Their description of community life in Greenwich Village reminded me of the fused characteristic of young-adult friendships. Since they had been together so long, their own love relationship maintained this joined quality. Like many relationships of people in the prime of young adulthood, their friendship was more like a "twinship."[1]

These were relationships formed during moments of developmental transition (Bodnar, 1992). They met in college. They discovered sexuality together. They supported each other through the difficult process of coming out to their families and friends. They spoke the same language, sometimes even completing each other's sentences. They both used the idiosyncratic term "Christmas balls" to refer to their tree ornaments. They had similar thought processes. Mr. M and his lover focused on details, not wholes. Their ideas were linear and not circular. They were known by family to have tempers. Mr. M was expressive. His lover expressed anger through silence and withdrawal. They shared aspects of each other's consciousness (Bakhtin, 1981; Vygotsky, 1967).

In the modern urban culture of the United States, most people, including homosexuals and lesbians, tend not to settle into solidified role relationships until their late 30s or early 40s. This being the case, the intimate relationships tend to be more fluid, with fewer boundaries. There is a natural and healthy merging of identities that is part of the growth process. In a culture that values ongoing self-improvement strategies, such as higher education, therapy, and other forms of sanctioned self-exploration, individuals tend to relate to each other in states of natural enmeshment for longer periods of time. Thus, young intimate friends tend to live with and through one another—they become parts of an organic whole.

I witnessed lovers become the functional minds for their demented partners. I observed intimate caretakers actually knowing what their loved one wanted or needed with few words being exchanged. I watched friends take over the professional tasks that couldn't be managed by the one who was ill. I saw loved ones actually assume the ill person's external role or identity.

The quality of individual relationships forming a whole was apparent on the AIDS unit. The MASH-like quality, the ongoing tragedy of continuous deaths, fostered a unique interdependence of people. They transcended traditional role relationships. Families were constituted of friends as well as blood relatives. People loved each other in many unique configurations that defied explanation. Often doctors, staff, and patients related like friends, with very little disruption to the work at hand, but sometimes they quarreled like enemies, with equally minimal disruption to the work. This tendency to construct a shared

1. This idea was put forth by Levinson (1978), who defined twinship as the sharing of a common dream. Mann (1985) put forth the notion that such friendships play an important role in the young adult's encounter with reality.

consciousness with friends seemed particular to AIDS work.[2]

A more personal construction of role relationships enabled a shared consciousness to evolve between patients and staff. The judicious use of intimacy fostered honesty and authenticity. The more personal construction of role relationships may have been possible because sexuality couldn't be taken for granted. The questioning of gender created many possibilities between the polarities of male and female. I felt released from the trap of a feminine identity. I could be powerful without losing the nurturing components of my personality. Patients and staff respected me, even when I displayed vulnerability. My authority, my expertise, and my knowledge didn't have to be won. Patients and staff simply weren't afraid to acknowledge competency in a woman. This freed me to explore the "multiple selves" (Mitchell, 1993) within myself and my patients. I recognized with them our shared consciousness, and the variety of ways there were to be a person.

Two men with cryptosporidiosis (a parasite that attacks the intestines and causes virulent diarrhea) shared a room. Mr. Q was a 40-year-old white banker with an Episcopalian background. Mr. F was a 23-year-old Hispanic male who worked as a manicurist. Mr. Q had a terrible depression and immediately disliked everyone. Mr. F, in addition to lymphoma, had HIV-induced mania. Initially they were often hospitalized together because neither was contagious to the other. Later they were hospitalized together because they couldn't be apart. Mr. F would often become overwhelmed and weep uncontrollably. Only Mr. Q could comfort him, with a robust, "Shut up, or I will never talk to you again!" Mr. Q couldn't sleep until Mr. F returned from his nightly rounds of fellow patients and staff. Mr. Q was terrified of being alone, and would often call out, "Are you there?" And Mr. F would sing something to him.

Once I overheard Mr. F call a nurse for Mr. Q. No one came. Someone was dying. An inexperienced intern had ordered life support on a patient who didn't wish to be artificially resuscitated. This provoked mayhem on the unit. Half the doctors were dutifully applying life-saving measures, and the other half were busy with outrage. Mr. F became urgent. Mr. Q was crying. His diaper was soiled, and the humiliation of his helplessness had finally eroded his stiff and tough exterior. So Mr. F did what any friend might do under the circumstances. He helped his friend change his diaper, in silence. My job was to close the door.

Other relational frontiers were also crossed. One young bisexual

2. I have also witnessed this solidarity, interdependence, and softer professional boundaries on child cancer units. In contrast, my experience on adult cancer units is that the professional boundaries are more rigid.

man, an executive in a major corporation, asked for help with his child. He was very close to death, living sometimes at home, sometimes in the hospital. His wife was stressed and tearful, and their three year-old daughter was deeply affected. She was reverting to the use of a bottle and a diaper. She was having nightmares. He felt strongly that he wanted to hold his daughter and comfort her. He wished her to remember her father's arms around her at a time when she really needed him. He was weak, though, and he had a tube coming out of his chest through which he could receive medication and nutritional supplements. He was afraid she would be terrified at the discovery of the tube and be traumatized. Our work together concentrated on introducing his daughter slowly to the machinery that was keeping her father alive. When he finally invited her into his bed and hugged her, she smiled. They curled up together.

As a psychologist in this environment, I pondered long and hard about boundaries. I wanted to impose more order and structure and to define roles clearly, until I understood the significance of interdependence. The only way to preserve the dignity of dying people was to fully acknowledge and legitimize their humanness, especially when they were at their most inhuman. To fully accomplish this, a doctor, nurse, or psychologist couldn't be resolutely professional. To do this implied that the entire existence of the other person in the relationship was contained in the patient role. To preserve the humanity of the last days or months of a person's life, the patient role had to be distributed evenly with the person's other roles: parent, child, lover, business person, socialite, writer, friend. The accepted redistribution of power in moments of death influenced me. Now I tolerate it all the time.

Dying

Mr. N was one of the few African-American gay men on the unit. He and I worked together twice-weekly for almost the entire year. He said that if it weren't for the fact that he was dying, he never would have gotten as close to a white woman as he had gotten to me. I was surprised and sorry to hear his feelings of dread when dealing with white people. I was less surprised to hear his discomfort when dealing with other African-Americans. Color difference didn't make him feel as insecure as sexual-orientation difference. He was a poet who had learned to play the guitar late in life. White to him was the color vanilla, the kind of ice cream his father had brought to his kids before he left home.

Mr. N used to sing the blues, and wanted to be Billie Holliday. He lay back in his hospital bed with soap-opera characters sobbing on the TV. Like a song, he recounted his early love of T, and how she threw him out when he lost his job for the first time. T was a college girl, and she wanted to be part of that frightening white world. She wasn't afraid to separate identity from skin color in the same way he was. He told me, "If all white people could be a little more black, they would love life a little bit more. If all black people would be a little more white, they would fear life just a little bit less."

As a young man, he used to crawl through a crevice in an abandoned building. The sunlight poured in through the chipped walls like crystal patterns. He rested back-to-back with his friend F while the heroin they just shot up made music from their breath. He thought it was sexy because he was high. It took him years to admit that he was attracted to men. He got high because he was afraid. He used his own racism to avoid a white society that was beginning to make room for homosexuals.

I was with him when he died. He was going into massive organ failure. We had our last conversation. He was happy to have known me. He suggested I find the time to be a poet. When he stopped breathing the next day, I watched life extinguish itself. His energy didn't seem to go anywhere. His life force was instantaneously absorbed by the atmosphere, the cosmos, or something. I knew that at least in memory, he would always be a part of me. Then I wondered why in death it is easier for people who are different to be a part of each other.

To the extent that psychology perpetuates the dualism of universality and particularism, it remains surprising that the ongoing tension between autonomy and interdependence in human nature inspires less interest in current theoretical trends (Fromm, 1941). I wonder if the loss of so many people will change the focus of psychoanalytic inquiry, or challenge the values of our culture. When would we evolve to a more transcendent exposition of our humanity? At times, I ranted. Anger cleansed my soul's palate.

In the meantime, Mr. R's illness worsened. His day planner lay next to his bed unopened. Quieter, he now refused further radiation treatment. Lucid moments were interspersed with delirium. He was terrified of the ants in his bed, the creatures that lurked in his room at night. It was Friday, and I had a feeling he might not be alive on Monday. He waited for me. "I knew you would be here," he whispered.

I smiled. "I came to say good-bye."

"I can tell by the stiffness of your grin you think this may be the final one."

I managed a somewhat truthful response, something like, "Yeah, I am afraid of that."

"Me too." Silence. "Could you cover my shoulders?" he asked.

By now, I was no longer following the tenets of psychotherapy as I had learned them in graduate school. On the AIDS unit, I had learned new rules. I pulled the soft blanket he had brought from home up higher over his shoulders, noting that he was trembling. He reached his arm as if to touch my forehead, but he wasn't strong enough, and sighed in his defeat. "No frowning."

I smiled and remembered when he first pointed out how often I frowned. He told me then, "Anger doesn't become you." He was so right. I had come to work on the AIDS unit a very angry young woman, only I hadn't realized it. Defiant and proud, I expressed my fury at life by working hard and burning away the edges of my joy. They were the reactions of a confused young widow who hadn't yet found her way in a world that didn't yet understand the impact of loss on young people.

At that moment, I had trouble finding words for this 33-year-old man with whom I had this relationship. A patient? A friend? Mr. R? Regular role relationships seemed inadequate when a person is dying.

"I don't know what to say," I told him. " I wonder if I've made you feel like a child."

"Your child?" he said with surprise.

"Maybe."

"Actually, Susan, I've always thought of you as my child. I've been putting all the parts of me that never had the chance to grow up inside of you so that they still can."

Conclusion

A few days after Mr. R died, I had what could loosely be termed a "session" with Mr. D. A 28-year-old man, he once had a wonderful career as a classical musician. He was also a comic. It was hard to know which he loved more. His friends recounted his brave attitude when he was diagnosed with HIV, and his attempts to keep his spirits high. A loving and generous man, he had always volunteered time to work with the sick and homeless. He was devastated when diagnosed with PML, and his lover was heartbroken. It was bad enough he could no longer play music. What would his life be like if he couldn't tell jokes? By the time I met him, the damage to his brain had resulted in his being paralyzed from the neck down. He knew his name, and he knew the names of friends, though he sometimes couldn't tell them apart. He knew the name of his disease. He talked in a strange tinkering monotone, but he was determined. Whenever I went to see him, he would say, "My name is D. Do you know a joke?" I always tried to find a new joke for him, even though I don't happen to be very funny. He knew. "Not funny, Susan, not funny."

Retaining some use of his right hand, he always said good-bye by lifting his hand and, with half-clenched fist, he would attempt to raise his thumb in the air. I knew him only a few weeks before his friends arranged for him to go to a house by the sea with the people he loved, for what would be the last weeks of his life. I wanted to say good-bye. I clumsily told him that I wasn't sure how much he understood. I wished him to know that he had inspired me, that I appreciated him.

"Is there anything, anything I can do at all for you?" I asked. "Is there anything I can do to say good-bye?"

Smiling, he raised his thumb and asked, "May I have this dance?"

I raised my thumb to his. The words floated in our gaze like choreography. I was swirling, and whirling, and waltzing across the floor.

My years working with persons who have AIDS propelled me forward to create a whole new life. In the field of psychology, we talk a great deal about the therapist-patient relationship. I have become convinced that therapist and patient are two extreme points in a continuum of role relationships. The work of psychoanalysis is to achieve balance. We don't have to articulate our patient selves, but we have to listen. We can hear our patient's efficacy when they show us their therapist selves—the strength and potential for healing they hold within their hearts. There is a dialectic in the therapeutic encounter. We respect it by allowing its motion.

Every person's life is a lens through which to experience an individual as an extension and a creator of his or her culture. A multiplicity of voices forms the consciousness of all persons. The people I have come to know are a part of me and I am a part of them.

My way of coping with so much loss of life was to listen carefully to what each person was discovering on his or her deathbed, and to tuck the wisdom away for safekeeping. My promise to most of the people with whom I worked was to share what I had learned about their lives. Their mistakes could be passed on to those who had yet to commit those same errors. Their deaths were in the name of a better life for others. I always said, "Plant your personality like seeds in a garden."

Living in the time of AIDS we are learning, I hope, to tend to the seeds that those we have loved and lost have planted within us. My memories are becoming flowers now. The way I work as a psychologist and as a psychoanalyst is an attempt to embody the models of authenticity, collaboration, and interdependence that have been taught to me by people who were dying, and by those who cared for the dying. Life is the love of dances.

References

Bakhtin, M. M. (1981), *The Dialogic Imagination,* ed. M. Holquist (trans. C. Emerson & M. Holquist). Austin: University of Texas Press.

Bodnar, S. (1992), Friendship and the Construction of the Person in Adult Development. Unpublished doctoral dissertation, City University of New York.

Fromm, E. (1941), *Escape from Freedom.* New York: Rhinehart.

Levinson, D. (1978), *The Seasons of a Man's Life.* New York: Knopf.

Mann, C. (1985), Adult development: Individuation, separation, and the role of reality. *Contemp. Psychoanal.,* 21:284–296.

Mitchell, S. (1993), *Hope and Dread in Psychoanalysis.* New York: Basic Books.

Vygotsky, L. S. (1967), *Thought and Language.* Cambridge, MA: MIT Press.

Index

A
Abandonment feelings, in dementia patient, 76
Abrams, D., 17, *57*
Abstinence, risk of, 50–51
Abuse, *See also* specific type of abuse
  of children of parents with AIDS, 83
Abuser, vicarious identification with, 197
Acting out, 147, 151
  after session, 149
  dissociation through, 158–159
  versus open relationship, 216–217
  refraining from, 153
  sexually compulsive, 155
Acting-out patient, sexually compulsive, 148
Activist groups, 57
ACT-UP, 100
Adjustment reaction with mixed emotions, 139, 140
Adler, G., 29, *57*
Adolescent, adolescence
  risk-taking during, 49
  sexuality, HIV-infected parent's fears related to, 90
Affect, release of, 148
Africa, AIDS in, 6, 12
Agazarian, Y. M., 182, *190*
  technique of, 182, 183
Aggression, sexual compulsivity and, 148–156
AIDS
  course of illness and medical treatment, 11–12
  different periods of, 15
  incidence of, 12
  knowledge on, gaps in, 15
  as leading cause of death, 82
  as payment for bad behavior, 185, 185
  protease inhibitors for, *See* Protease inhibitors
  as punishment, 201
  sources of information on, xviii
  stages of, 52
  survivors of, *See* Survivors
  symptomatic, onset of, 7
  syphilis and, 52–54
  transmission of, rate of, 53
  treatment of, *See* Treatment
AIDS crisis, 99–100
AIDS epidemic, psychological aspects of
  after the cure, 54–57
  AIDS and syphilis, 52–54
  bereavement, 29–36, *See also* Bereavement
  choice of issues to work on, 21–24
  course of illness and medical treatment, 11–12
  cultural determinants in AIDS issues, 47–48
  historical overview, 4–11
  HIV testing and AIDS anxiety, 42–44

AIDS epidemic, psychological aspects of *(continued)*
HIV testing and confidentiality, 45–46
HIV-negative patients, 39–42
initial diagnosis, 17–19
in late-stage AIDS, 24–25
learning of HIV-positive diagnosis, 14–17
loneliness and, 25–26
negotiating safer sex, 48–52
psychotherapist in, 26–29, *See also* Psychotherapist
psychotherapy with AIDS patient, goals and countertransference, 12–14
suicidal ideation, 37–38
survivor guilt, 36–37
timing of interpretations, 19–21
unconscious factors in assessing one's risk for HIV, 46–47
unsafe sex and lying to partners, 38–39
AIDS organizations, 167
AIDS patients
working with, xix
stigma associated with, xviii
AIDS-related complex (ARC), 52
AIDS Treatment News, 15
AIDS unit, inpatient, staff
coping with AIDS, 222–223
losses in, 224
Ailments, trivial, seeking treatment for, 211n
AL-721, 9
Alcoholics Anonymous, 91
Aliveness, 189
Allopathic treatments, 127
Alternative communities, construction of, 99
Alternative treatments, 17, 115, 116, 122, 123
Altman, N., xixn, *xxiv*
Altruism, 75
Altschul, S., 82, *94*
Amaro, H,, 50, *58*
Ambivalence, in children of parents with AIDS, 84–85
reconciliation of, 85
Americans, unpreparedness for dealing with prospect of dying, 76–77
Anal intercourse
HIV transmission by, myths related to, 8
literature on, government refusal of funding for, 8–9
use of condom during, 50
Anderson, J.B., 175, *190*
Andrea del Sarto (Browning), xix
Anger
toward death of group member, 179
expressed through silence and withdrawal, 229
loss of, 10
as motive for living, 186
in sexually compulsive gay man, 155
toward therapist, seroconversion during psychotherapy and, 202, 205
Anxiety, 20
HIV
pathologic, psychoanalytic interpretation for, 42
syndrome of "depression" secondary to, 41
HIV testing and, 42–44
reactive, 134
Appointment
cancellations, 148
keeping of, 141, 150
missed, 147–148
Aronson, S., 83, 92, *94*
Art, pervasive presence of AIDS in, 53
Assertiveness, 201, 202
seroconversion during psychotherapy and, 204
Atkinson, J.H., 53, *58*
Atmosphere, therapeutic, 66

Attachment
hiatuses in, 86
of HIV-infected parent, to children, 89–90
new, child's formation of, 87
Auerbach, J., 40, *58*
Authenticity, 230
Authorities, acceptance by, 70
Authority, use of, 225
Autoeroticism, 151–152
Autonomy, 232
restoring of, 68–69
Avoidance, physical, 67
Azim, H. F. A., 212, *219*
AZT, 16
avoidance of, 126
treatment of mother, transmission of HIV to child and, 48

B

Baba, T., 51, *58*
Bactrim, 12
Badness, 185, 185n
Bakhtin, M.M., 229, *235*
Barbiturates, stockpiling of, 38
Bayer, P., 21, *58*
Beckett, A., 183, 186, *190*
Behavior, *See also* specific type of behavior
HIV transmission related to, 8
Beiser, M., 29, *57*
Belief system, AIDS-related, 7–8
Bell-ringing, structured, 227
Belongings, disposal of, 171
Benjamin, J., 199, *207*
Bereavement, 29–31, *See also* Mourning
childhood, 82, 85, *See also* Children, of parents with AIDS
chronic, 164, *See also* Chronic loss and grief
ventilation of feelings about, 164
as countertransference problems, 33–34
extent of, listening to, 165
massive, 31–36
Bereavement groups, *See also* Gay men's bereavement group
short term, 212
BETA: Bulletin of Experimental Treatments for AIDS, 15
Bey, M., 48, *58*
Bion, W.R., 212, *219*
Bisexual men, AIDS in, 12
Bitterness, 185
Black death, 32
Blaming, 19
Blechner, M. J., xix, xx, *xxiv*, 6, 13, 24, 31, 56, *58*, 218, *219*
Blindness, 24
Blood products, transfer of, 7
Blood supply, inadequate testing and monitoring, 9
Bloom, J., 24, *62*
Boccaccio, G., 32, *58*
Bodily cleansing, 17
Bodnar, S., 229, *235*
Body fluids, transfer of, 7
Boswell, J., 201, *207*
Boundaries, on AIDS unit, 231
Bowel accidents, 171
Bowlby, J., 82, *94*
Boyer, P., 48, *59*
Breast cancer, activist groups, 57
Brief therapeutic encounters, 105
Brodie, H., 40, *58*
Browning, F., 196, *207*
"journey of difference" and, 196
Browning, R., xix
Bryson, Y., 48, *59*
Buchbinder, S., 12n, 13n, 14, 51, *58, 60, 61*
Burch, B., 216, *219*

C

Callen, M., 28, *58*
Cancer victims, activist groups, 57
Candidiasis, oral, 11
Cannon, L., 51, *60*
Cao, Y., 12n, *58*

Capitanio, J., 8, 60
Career
concerns related to, 123, 125
setbacks, 211
Caretaker
new, for children of parents with AIDS
collateral work for, 92
new, of children of parents with AIDS, transfer of positive feelings and attachment to, 85–86
Caretaking, unresolved guilt about, 30
Caretaking roles, usurping of, 211
Catania, J., 39, *60*
Catholic Church, condemnation of homosexuality, 138
Catholicism, 135
Caucasians, genetic anomaly for resistance to AIDS, 13n
Centers, services to AIDS families, 93
Centers for Disease Control (CDC), 82, 93, *94*
definition of AIDS, 7
Chancre sores, 6
Channeling, 127
Chappell, M., 134, *142*
Character resistances, confrontation of, 18
Character traits, working on, judgments for, 21–22
Chatelaine, K., xx, *xxv*
Chi Kung exercises, 146, 151
Child abuse, 198
Childhood history, difficulty with intimacy and, 99
Children
boarding care for, 82
of parents with AIDS, 81–82, 188
alternative types of treatment modalities, 92–93
ambivalence toward parent, 88
future of, 93–94
issues and themes in grief work with, 83–87
scope of problem, 82–83
treatment considerations, 87–92
underserved, 82–83
of substance-using parents, neglect of, 84
Chinese cucumber, 9
Choices, 150
Christianity, 201
Chronic loss and grief, 210, 212
managing of, case study, 163–165
background, 165
beginning of psychotherapy, 167–169
losses, 165–167
therapeutic relationship in, 171–172
in transference and countertransference, 172–174
use of psychotherapy, 169–171
Chumship, creating of, 102
Close discourse, 107
Closeness
fear of, 24
sharing of, with group leader, 182
Clothing, dreams of, 124
Coates, T., 39, *60*
Cognitive deficits, 12, 53
Cohen, O., 12n, *61*
Cole, R., 29, *57*
College students, heterosexual, practice of safer sex by, 48–49
"Coming out," 211, 228
Communication
blocks in, 33
open, 88, 90, 91
Community meetings, 101
Compulsive behavior, 75
Condom, use of, 50
effects of, 198–199
male attitude toward, 50
Confidence, loss of, 68

Confidentiality
absolute, necessary changes in, 72
HIV testing and, 45–46
loss of, fear of, 71
for prisoners, 98
Conflict, internal, 151
Confrontation, 108
Connor, E., 48, *58*
Consciousness, shared, 229–230
"Contact victimization," 172
Contagion, fear of, xviii, 19, 121
Control
loss of, 141
need for, 71, 201
rebelling against, 200–201
Coping resources, depleted, 211
Counseling, pretest and posttest, 46
Countertransference, *See also* Transference-countertransference
analysis of, xxiii, 19
in suicidal ideation, 38
complementary to, 16
death and mortality and, 28
group leader's, 188
disease and death and, 188–190
sexual orientation and, 188
during psychotherapy of young HIV-positive woman, case study, 115–130
radical, 218
traumatic, 172
unsafe sex and lying to partner and, 39
use in psychotherapy of AIDS patient, 13–14
Countertransference explorations, in HIV-positivity development during psychotherapy, 197
Countertransference problems
about loss, 164
in treating HIV-positive drug abusers, 100–101
County department of health, HIV testing by, 45
Couples counseling, 103
Coupling, 217
Courtois, C., 172, *174*
Crack addict, traits of, 111
Cryptosporidiosis, 230
Culture
acceptance of death and, 76
AIDS issues and, 47–48
antihomosexual bias in, 74
determinants of AIDS issues, 47–48
symbolic meaning of AIDS and syphilis and, 53
Cure for AIDS, 14, 131
fantasies on, 24–25
issues following, 54
illusion of man's ability to conquer disease, 55
need for social change, 55–56
value of psychotherapy for other serious physical diseases, 56–57
Curiosity, 106
Cytomegalovirus, 11, 24

D

Daniolos, P., 39, *58*
Dansky, S., 25, *59*
Dating workshops, 103
Davies, P., 50, *59*
Death and dying, 12
on AIDS unit, 231–233
avoidance of topic, 28, 178
denial of, 116, 130
discussion of, in group process, 184
emotions surrounding, 78
fear of, 103–1104
first, in group, 179–180
discussion of, by leader, 180, 181
group leader's countertransference and, 188–190
incidence of, 12, 12n
patient close to, adaptation of

Death and dying *(continued)*
psychotherapy for, 109–110
psychologist associated with, 108
theoretical models of, 28
uncertain but close, panic of, 24
Death rate, AIDS-related, 209
Death wish, expression of, in sexual behavior, 151
Decameron, The (Bocaccio), 32
Decision, decision making
delicate, therapist's making of, 75
by patient, 68, 69
Defense(s), 71
in group process, 189
interpreting and supporting of, 18
against safer sex, 49
Defensive meaning, 22
Delusions, in repeat survivors, 32–33
Demarest, B., 12n, *61*
Dementia, AIDS, 12, 109
case study, 133–142
dealing with, 75–76
history in, 135–137
course of treatment and questions related to, 137–142
therapist's functions in, 24
Denial, 6, 44, 71
defense of HIV testing and, 42
need for, 108
in patient with dementia, 139–140
in patient's dreams, 34
projected, 41
in repeated survivors, 33
of seriousness of illness, 179
Dependency, conflicts related to, 227
Depression
chronic, 134
reactive, 134
related to chronic loss and grief, 173
in repeated survivors, 33
seroconversion during
psychotherapy and, 202, 204
in sexually compulsive gay man, 158
in surviving partner, 30
syndrome of, 41
treatment for, refusal of, 226
Deprivation, in children of parents with AIDS, 92
Despair, 185
versus creative commitment to life, 183–185
guiltless, 184n
Deveikis, A., 48, *59*
Developmental vacuum, 86
Diagnosis
HIV-positive, patient's learning of, counseling for, 14–17
initial, patient's psychotherapeutic efforts in, 17–19
issues of, 109
Dialogue, *See also* specific type of dialogue
therapeutic, patient's entry into, 66
Dickover, R., 48, *59*
Diet, 121, 122
Different, sense of being, 215
Dimen, M., 216, *219*
Discomfort, 64
Disease
group leader's countertransference and, 188–190
illusion of man's ability to conquer, 55
Disgrace, in HIV patient, 69
Displacement, 5
Dissociation, through drug abuse and acting out, 158–159
Distortion, in AIDS epidemic, 5
Doctor, *See also* Physician; therapist
good, 104
Domanski, M., 48, *59*
Domarus, E. von, 8, *59*
principle of, 8
Domestic violence, 98
Domination, desire for, 201

Dora case, 54
Dream(s)
  in AIDS anxiety, 43–44
  of death, 184
  denial and reaction formation in, 34
  of group leader, 189
  in identity confusion, 124
  related to impact of multiple losses, 224
  seroconversion during psychotherapy-related, 197–198, 206
  in sexually compulsive gay man, 158
  unresolved conflicts in, 28
  on unsafe sex, 51–52
Drescher, J., xix, *xxv*
Dualism, 232
Dying people, *See also* Death and dying
  dignity of, preserving of, 231

E
Early intervention, patient's decision for, 16–17, 17n
Education, of young, about HIV, 49
Egan, D., 48, *59*
Ego defenses, 5
Ehrhardt, A., 50, *59*
Eisold, B. K., 188, *190*
Eissler, K., 29, *59*
Ejaculation, difficulty in, 137, 138
Elashoff, R., 24, *59*
Emmerich, A., 93, *94*
Emotion, 155
  expression of, 26–27
  primary, 108
Empathy, 173
  blocks to, 28
  failure in, 218
  gaining of, 42
Energy, in group members, 184, 184n
Engel, R., 51, *61*
European Collaborative Study, 48, *59*
Exploitation, 22

F
Fahey, J., 24, *59*
"Falling off the wagon," 50
Family
  assurances from, 165
  displacement of lover, 211, 212
  extended, connection of child to parent with AIDS, 87
  informing and involving of, 73
  rage in, 84, 86–87
  single, child of parent with AIDS raised in, 85
Fantasy, 154
  about self, 107
  of becoming HIV-positive, 194
  of being infected, in children of parents with AIDS, 86
  expression of, 26–27
  idealizing, 194
  interpretation of, 158
  seroconversion during psychotherapy and, 202, 206
  suicidal, 37–38, *See also* Suicidal ideation
Far discourse, adaptation of psychotherapy for, 105–106, 107
Father, *See also* Parent
  difficulties with, 215–216
Fatigue, 146
Fauci, A., 12n, *61*
Fawzy, F., 24, *59*
Fawzy, N., 24, *59*
Fear, 5, 67
  of AIDS, 8, 40, 41, 42, 43
    cultural differences in, 47–48
    dissociated, 41
    excessive, 44
    manifestly inadequate, 46
    unconscious or acknowledged, 40–41, 44, 46
  of becoming gravely ill and helpless, 184

Fear *(continued)*
in children of parents with AIDS, 86
in HIV-infected parent, of infecting child, 91
reality-based, 173
Fee, higher, patient's response to, 168
Ferenczi, S., 18, *59*, 130
Fetus, transmission of HIV to, viral load and, 48
Financial policies, limitation of role of psychotherapy by, 63
Fiscalini, J., xxiv, *xxv*
Fishman, B., 42, *61*
Follmann, D., 48, *59*
Fonagy, P., 86, *94*
Forgetfulness, in patient with dementia, 139, 140
Fraiberg, S., 90, *94*
Frances, A., 42, *61*
Frank, A., 93, *94*
Fraternal conflict, 195–196, 198
Freud, A., 93, *94*
Freud, S., 5, 18, 30, *59*
concept of wish-fulfillment, 4
strategy for interpretation, 20n
thoughts about death and health, 130
thoughts on rich and fulfilling life, 131
view on syphilis, 54
Friends
assurances from, 165
loyalty to, 169
Fromm, E., 232, *235*
Fromm-Reichmann, F., xxv, *xxv*
"Full-blown-AIDS," 52
Function, loss of, 171
Funeral plans, making of, 211, 212
by patient, 142
Furman, E., 83, *94*

G

Gabriel, M. A., 179, 181, *190*
Gardens, 183
Garraty, E., 48, *59*
Gay cotherapist, for gay men's bereavement group, 212–213
Gay doctor, feelings of, 77–78
Gay man, 6, 12
with AIDS, children of, 188
experiences in heterosexual world, 213
HIV-negative, isolation from, 22
HIV-positive
multiple losses in, *See* Chronic loss and grief
sense of belonging, 22
sexually compulsive, *See* Sexually compulsive HIV-positive gay man
monogamous relationships in, 55–56, 56
safer sex and, 50
young, safety from HIV infection, false beliefs related to, 7
Gay marriage, legitimizing of, 55, 56
Gay men's bereavement group, heterosexual male therapist's self-discovery in, case study, 209–214
monogamy: acting out versus open relationship, 216–217
political and personal: continuous or separate realities, 217–219
sexual identity: learned versus innate, 214–216
Gay Men's Health Crisis (GMHC), 167, 169, 176
Geertz, C., 102, *112*
Gelber, R., 48, *58*
Gender identity, *See also* Sexual identity
struggle with, 98
Gender-role-related behaviors, delineation of, 188
Gerber, M., 20n, *59*
"Getting used to" AIDS, 33
Giorgi, J., 12n, *61*
GMHC *Newsletter of Experimental AIDS Therapies*, 15
Goals

appropriate, 131
patient's, 23
God
as protector, 201
relationship to, 204
Gold, J., 42, *61*
Goldman, S., 32, *60*
Gottheil, E., 24, *62*
Government, irrationality related to AIDS epidemic, 8–9
Gox, C., 12n, *61*
Grandparents, as caretaker for children of parents with AIDS, 87
Graniosi, C., 12n, *61*
Grant, I., 53, *58*
Graves, R., 20, *60*
Green, J., 21, 56, *60*
Greenberg, J., 17, *60*
Greene, M., 51, *58*
GRID (Gay-Related Immune Disorder), 4
Grief, 78
in children of parents with AIDS, 92
chronic, *See* Chronic loss and grief
dealing with, 29
in HIV-negative partner, 32
resolution, 87
seroconversion during psychotherapy and, 202
in therapist, 34–35, 202
Grieving, continued, 212
Group(s), *See also* Group process; Group therapy
leaving of, rage and, 186–187
patient's joining of, 72
Group leader
neutrality and anonymity, 212–213, 214
rage at, 187
Group process, from psychodynamic point of view, case study, 175–176
choosing members, 176–178
countertransference, 188–190, *See also* Countertransference
early definition of group purpose, 178
first death, 179–180
members' experience: life on fast-forward versus despair, 183–185
rage and, 185–187
role of group leader, 180–183
Group programs, substance abuser's work in, 110
Group therapy, 206
change to, 73
for children of parents with AIDS, 92
for gay men's bereavement, *See* Gay men's bereavement group
for relief of shame, 70
Guilt, 185
religious, related to homosexuality, 138
survival, 36–37, 211
denial of, 36–37
in repeated survivors, 33
unresolved, 30
Gunther, H. C., xxiv, *xxv*
Gupta, P., 10, *61*
Guthrie, D., 24, *59*

H

Haitians, 6
Hallucinations
in repeat survivors, 32–33
in surviving partner, 30, 31
Hands-on-healing techniques, 124–125
Harris, A., 216, *219*
Hate, 205
Hausman, K., 8, *60*
Havens, J., 82, 93, *94*
Hay, L., 10
Healers, 122
Healing crisis, 125
Healing Wise (Weed), 123
Health, therapist's inquiries regarding, 119

Heckler, M., 6
Help, patients need to provide, 108
Helplessness feelings, 189
  in therapist, 202
Hemophiliacs, 6, 9, 12
Henig, R.M., 53, *60*
Hepatitis B, 202, 203
Herbal remedies, 123
Herek, G., 8, *60*
Herman, J. L., 172, *174*
Herman, S., 48, *59*
Herpes infections, 11
Heschel, A. J., 104, *112*
Hessol, N., 51, *60, 61*
"Heterosexism," 212
Heterosexuals, HIV-infected, 6, 12
High meaning, 22–23
High-risk behavior, 193
  in HIV-negative partner, 194
Hillman, J., 100, *112*
Hirsch, I., 218, *219*
History, early, exploration of, 27–28
HIV Center for Clinical and Behavioral Studies Report, 6n, *60*
HIV (human immunodeficiency virus) infection, 5, 52, 193
  approach to, polarities of, 50
  latency period of, 7
  medical treatment of, 12
  misconceptions related to, 6
  natural resistance to, 7
  nonprogression of, 7
  progression to AIDS, 6, 12, 12n, 14
  resistance to, 13n
  spread of, prevention of, 74
  test for antibodies to, 5
  transmission, prevention of, 48, *See also* Safer sex
HIV (human immunodeficiency virus)-negative patients, 5
  HIV-related issues in, 39–42
  "worried well," 5–6
HIV (human immunodeficiency virus)-positive patient
  first-encounter with, 67
  infection of others, 74
  life of
    damage inflicted on, 64
    external realities of, 64
  unsafe sex and lying to partner, 38–39
HIV (human immunodeficiency virus)-positive status
  changes related to, 116
  life centered around, 124
  patient's lack of knowledge of, 49, 49n
  refusal of disclosure
    to physician, 128
    to sexual partner, 128
  revealing of, consequences of, 45–46
HIV (human immunodeficiency virus) test, 42
  AIDS anxiety and, 42–44
  confidentiality and, 45–46
  fear of, 50
  procrastination in taking, 40
  refusal of, 44, 166
  timing for, 41
Ho, D., 12n, *58*
Hoffman, I. Z., 218, *219*
Holistic practices, 17, 121, 146
Holmberg, S., 13n, 14, *58*
Holmes, V., 39, *58*
Holocaust, parallels with, 34
Home
  group leader's visit to, 180, 182
  patient's, treatment in, 76
  physical layout of, 176
Home aides, 135
Home test kit, 45
Homeopathic remedies, 17
Homophobia, 74–75, 166, 194, 214
  in family of homosexual, 87, 196
  internalized, 30, 69
  psychoanalysts training and, xix
  related to HIV transmission, 8
  therapist's, 212
  view of effeminate son, society and, 215
Homosexuality, *See also* Gay

conflicts related to, 227
problematic history of psychoanalysis with, xix
"Homosexuality equals psychopathology," 215
Honesty, 102, 230
Hope, 6, 178
loss of, 10
Hopelessness, 103
Hospital visits, by group leader, 182
Hospitalization, arrangement for, 182
HPA-23, 9
HTLV-III test, 145
Hugging, patient's request for, 67, 68
Human immunodeficiency virus, *See* HIV
Humanness, issue of, in treatment of sexually compulsive HIV-positive gay man, 146–148
Humor, approach to AIDS epidemic with, 34
Hyun, C., 24, *59*

I

Identification
problems in, in children of parents with AIDS, 86–87
vicarious, 197
Identity confusion, 124
Identity issues, 142
Ignorance, 8, 121
Imaging techniques, 17
Imber-Black, E., 91, *94*
Immune system
capacity of, markers for, 10
destruction of, 12
Impotence, 137, 138
Impulsive behavior, 75
Incest survivor, sexually compulsive, treating of, 150
Individual psychotherapy, 73
adaptation of, 105
to difficult patient population, 105–108
to patients with extended life spans, 108–109
when someone is close to death, 109–110
self-image improvement by, 70
Infections, sexual, minor, 37
Information collector, group leader as, 182
Insights, interpreting with, 18
Integration, 104–105
Interdependence, 232
Internist, need of feedback, 72
Interpersonal communication in dementia, 75
Interpersonal network, narrowing of, 164, 166
Interpersonal psychoanalysis
principles of, xxiii–xxiv
working with AIDS and, 13, 14
Interpersonal relations, survival of, 29
Interpretations, timing of, 19–21
Interview, initial, 65–66
Intimacy, 152, 229
flights from, 217
need for, 71
patient's difficulty with, 99
symbolic, 152
Intravenous (IV) drug abusers, 6, 12
detox program for, 55
fear of AIDS in, 48
Irrationality, related to AIDS, 8
Irrelevant meaning, 22
Isay, R. A., xix, *xxv*, 215, *219*
Isolation feelings, 178, 194, *See also* Loneliness
Iwasaki, T., 31, *62*

J

Jacobsberg, L., 42, *61*
Jealousy, parental, 90
Jeffrey, 50
Jewish mourning laws, 36, 36n
Johnston, L., 29, *57*

Johnston, W., 51. *60*
"Journey of difference," 196

K
Kaposi's sarcoma, 4, 11
  shame related to, 158
Karel, R., 8, *60*
Katz, M., 13n, 14, *58*
Keane, T., 93, *94*
Kegeles, S., 39, *60*
Keller, M., 48, *59*
Kerby, J. L., 175, *190*
Kernberg, O., 17, *60*
Kidney, malfunction, depression related to, 225
KIDS (film), 49
King, P., 17, *60*
Kingsley, L., 10, *61*
Kirp, D., 89, *95*
Kiselev, P., 48, *58*
Klein, M., 53, *60*
Koch, J., 51, *58*
Kohut, H., 184n, *190*
  view on guiltless despair, 184n
Kraemer, H., 24, *62*
Krant, M., 29, *57*
Kübler-Ross, E., 26, 28, 29, 57, *60*, 188, *190*

L
Lamm, M., 36n, *60*
Language, use of, 155
Late-stage AIDS
  loneliness in, 25–26
  psychotherapy with patients in, 24–25
Laudry, C. P., 175, *190*
Legionnaire's disease, 9
Legislation, gay rights, 210
Levenson, E., 218, *219*
Levine, C., 82, *95*
Levinson, D., 229n, *235*
  definition of twinship, 229n
Lewes, K., xix, *xxv*
Life
  creative commitment to, versus despair, 183–185
  review of, 184, 185
  saving of, 225–227
Life expectancy, in HIV-infected patients, 12, 12n
Life span, extended, patients with, adaptation of psychotherapy for, 108–109
Life-and-death issues, 142
Lifestyle
  losing of, 210
  therapist's willingness to deal with, 64
  unusual, revealing of, 66
Lifson, A., 51, *60*
Liminality, 99–100, 103
Limits, 108
Lindemann, E., 83, 84, *95*
Lionells, M., xxiv, *xxv*
Living, strategy for, 15
Locker, A., 82, 93, *94*
Loewald, H., 84, 86, *95*
Loneliness feelings, 25–26, 135
  period for, 26
  politics and, 217–218
Longtime Companion, 33
Loss
  chronic, *See* Chronic loss and grief
  dealing with, 29, *See also* Bereavement
  fall in status as, 210–212
  multiple and ongoing, 212, *See also* Multiple losses
Louie, L., 13n, 14, *58*
Love, romantic, 131
Lymphoma, AIDS-related, 227

M
Mania, HIV-induced, 230
Mann, C., xxiv, *xxv*, 229n, *235*
  definition of twinship, 229n
Mann, D., 13n, 14, *58*
Margolick, J., 12n, *61*
Marriage, 40, 55
  gay

legitimizing of, 56
monogamous, 55
society and, 55–56
for HIV-positive female, 122–123
Marris, P., 31, *60*
Maslow, A., 20n, *60*
Masochist, need for recognition, 199
Massage, 17
Masturbation, 50, 151, 154
Maximally avoidant approach to HIV infection and risk reduction, 50
Maximally permissive approach to HIV infection and risk reduction, 50
McCallum, M., 212, *219*
McCann, I. L., 172, *174*
McCutchan, J., 17, *60*
McLaughlin, S., 93, *94*
Meaning
of AIDS, conflicting, 22
shared system of, 102
Meaning-making, 22–23
Medical administration, limitation of role of psychotherapy by, 63
Medical considerations, in HIV-infected parents, 92
Medical establishment, patient's meshing with, 168
Medical expertise, discussion of, in group process, 178
Medical knowledge, therapist's, 13
Medical personnel, patient's relationship with, 177–178
Medical power of attorney, assigning of, 127
Medical protocols, discussion of, in group process, 178
Medical treatment, *See also* specific treatment
alternative, *See* Alternative treatment
conventional, 180
patient's participation in, 15
tracks for, 11–12
Medications, stockpiling of, 38
Mellins, C., 82, 93, *94*
Mellors, J., 10, *61*
Memorial services, planning of, 211, 212
Memory, 4
loss, 139, 140
Men, *See also* Gay man
unprotected vaginal intercourse in, chance of HIV infection by, 40
Mental health community, attention to AIDS, 53
Menzo, S., 12n, *61*
Metal lollipops, homeopathic, 125, 126
Mirroring, 50
Mitchell, S., xxiv, *xxv*, 230, *235*
Mittler, E., 51, *58*
Monette, P., 10n, 28, *61*
Monogamy, 55
breaks with, 217
overvaluation of, 216–217
Montefiori, D., 12n, *61*
Mood, shifts in, 202
Mood disorder, 75, 226
Mortality, *See* Death and dying
Morton, D., 24, *59*
Mother
intrusive, 216
overprotective, 216
Motivation, exploration of, 198
Mourning, *See also* Bereavement
analysis of transference and, 84
in children of AIDS patient, 84
chronic, 164
by group leader, 190
manifestations in children, 92
Multiple losses, 170, *See also* Chronic loss and grief
anger related to, 179
effect on group leader, 190
forms of, 210–212
grief related to, 212
impact on practice of psycho-

Multiple losses *(continued)*
analytically informed psychotherapy, case study, 221–223
dying and, 221–223
relationships in, 227–231
saving life, 225–227
upon entering the field, 222–224
integrating of, 163
isolation feelings related to, 194
massive bereavement related to, 31–32
personal network narrowing by, 164, 166
present, reverberation to past losses, 173
realization of, 171
survivor guilt and depression in, 33
therapist's responses to, 173
Myers, W., 17, *61*
Myth(s), about AIDS, 5, 7
Mythical figures, naming complexes and syndromes after, 20–21

N

Nagera, H., 86, *95*
Narcissism, 182n, 183n
Narcotics Anonymous, 91
National Commission on AIDS, 8
Needle
clean, ready access to, 8
-exchange programs, 9
Nervous system, HIV attack of, 12
Network, interpersonal, narrowing of, 164, 166
Neuropsychiatric functioning, HIV and, 53
Neutrality, weight of, freedom from, 214
New Age gurus, 10n
New relationship, hiding of, 36
New York Native, viii
New York Times, 9
Newsletters, on latest findings in AIDS, 15
Nichols, S. E., 183, 186, *190*
"Normal," desire to be, 128
Not-me attitude, 4, 5, 6, 9, 106
Not-me experience, 106
Note taking, 223–224
Nuland, S. B., 53, *61*
Nutritional regimens, 17

O

Object loss, 82
Object relations
bereavement and, 29
early, 198
promoting of, 86
Observational stance, 104
Odets, W., 51, *61*
Oedipal theory, 215
Oedipus complex, 20n
Okonogi, K., 31, *62*
O'Malley, P., 51, *60*
Open relationships, acting out versus, 216–217
Opportunistic infection, 11, 134
prophylaxis, 15
Oral sex, 50
Orenstein, J., 12n, *61*
Osborn, J., 8, *61*
O'Sullivan, M., 48, *58*
"Otherness," 101
Outside agencies, work with, 87

P

Packing, dreams of, 124
Pain, fear of, 24
Panic, 5, 44
Pantaleo, G., 12n, *61*
Parallel playing, 151
Parent, *See also* Father; Mother
with AIDS, children of, *See* Children
avoidance of recognition of homosexual orientation, 196
dead, identification with, 86
HIV-infected, attachment to children, 89

informing of HIV-positivity, 203–204
substance-abusing, risk of contracting HIV in, 82
Parental substitute, for children of parents with AIDS, 87
Parenting, troubled, homosexual causing, 215
Pares-Avila, J., 93, *94*
Particularism, 232
Partner
deceased, parents of, attitude toward surviving partner, 30–31
of HIV-positive patient, protection of, 74
lying to, about HIV status, 38–39
surviving, eviction from home, 30–31
therapist's need to work with, 72
Passivity, 108
Patient, blaming of, for illness, 19
Patient population, difficult, adaptation of psychotherapy to, 105–108
Patient role, 104
Paul (Saint), 50
Pearlman, L. A., 172, *174*
Peer counselors, substance abusers as, 109–110
Peer relations, 103
Penicillin, 55
Penninck, D., 51, *58*
Perception, 4
Performance anxiety, 107
"Permanency-planning" movement, 88
Perry, S. W., 42, *61*
Person, E. S., 188, *191*
Personal experience, losing of, 100
Personal life, versus political life, 217–219
Personality, undistinguished manifestations, 111
Personality styles, patient-physician, 15–16
Philadelphia, 46
Phone sessions, 127, 148
Physical contact, in HIV-positive patient, need for, 23
Physical illness, value of psychotherapy for, 56–57
Physician
burnout, 16
gay, *See* Gay doctors
organization of first response to AIDS crisis, 222
private, anonymous HIV testing by, 45
psychology of, 16
Piper, W. E., 212, *219*
Pizzo, P., 48, *59*
Plaeger, S., 48, *59*
Pneumocystis carinii pneumonia, 11, 15
onset of, forestalling of, 12
Politics, personal life and, 217–219
Pollack, G., 86, *95*
Porcelain doll feeling, 200
Postponing of issue, 71
Postrebound period, loneliness in, 26
Potential, unfulfilled, 111
Power, redistribution of, on AIDS unit, 231
Practical problems, dealing with, 170
Praying, following seroconversion, 204
Precautions, unnecessarily strict, 91
Pregnancy, in HIV-positive woman, 48
dangers of, 129
Prejudice, 8
removal of, xix
Press, coverage of AIDS, historical perspective, 9
Pressure, patient's experience of, 75
"Pressure-cooker" analysis, 19
Primary processes, 5
Prisoner, drug-abusers, treatment of, 98
Private testing facilities, anonymous testing in, 45

Probing, 70–72
Progressive multifocal leukoencephalopathy (PML), 134, 135, 137
"Projective interpretation," 24
Prostate cancer, mental health services for, 57
Protease inhibitors, 10, 11
  side effects of, 11
Proximal level, people engaging at, adaptation of psychotherapy for, 106–107
Psychic afterlife, 29
Psychic surgery, 126–127
Psychoanalysis
  practice of, denial of death in, 130
  therapeutic action of, xxiii
Psychoanalytic technique, elasticity of, 18
Psychoanalytically oriented treatment, xx1
Psychological knowledge, therapist's, 13
Psychological mindedness, change in, 23
Psychological ministrations, for AIDS treatment, failure of, 10, 10n
Psychologist, *See also* Therapist
  good or superior, 111
Psychopathology, 54, 82
  adaptive, 168
Psychosis, 53
Psychosomatic diseases, 130
Psychotherapeutic methods, modifying of, when treating HIV-positive patient, 63–65, 79
  art of probing, 70–72
  dealing with dementia, 75–76
  initial interview, 65–55
  relieving shame, 69–70
  restoring patient's autonomy and self-direction, 68–69
  therapist as moral policeman, 74–75
  therapist's special listening, 66
  therapist's touching and hugging, 67–68
  unaccustomed roles for therapist, 72–73
Psychotherapist, *See* Therapist
Psychotherapy
  with AIDS patient, goals and countertransference, 12–14
  deferring of, to medical needs, 226
  dementia and, 133, *See also* Dementia
  entering of, as sexual act, 150
  patient becoming HIV-positive during, case study, 193–206
  patient's relevance to, questioning of, 138
  patient's use of, in managing chronic grief and loss, 169–171
  reasons for seeking, 23
  role of, limiting of, 63
  traditional, time required for, 64
  value of
    in managing chronic loss and grief, 172
    for serious physical illnesses, 56–57
Push (Sapphire), 84
PWAs (People with AIDS), 180

Q

Qin, L., 12n, *58*
Questions, *See also* Probing
  asking of, by patient, 177
  central, in HIV-positive patient, 120
  patient's resistance to answering of, 71

R

Rabkin, J., 69, *79*
Race, 136
  IV drug use and, 12
  transmission of HIV and, 5
Racker, H., 218, *219*

Rage, 185
in children of patents with AIDS, 83–84, 88
at group leader, 187
at HIV status, 39
in parents with AIDS, 90
Rank, O., 18, *59*
Reaction formation, 4, 5
in patient's dreams, 34
Reagan, R., 9
Reality
contact with, diminishing of, 171
interpretation of, 158
Reality issues, confronting of, 103–104
Reanalysis, of group leader, reaction to death and, 189, 189n
Reasoning, 4
Recognition, need for, 199
Rees, W.D., 31, *61*
Rejection, moral, 67
Relapse, 75
Relatedness, style of, 20
Relational psychoanalysis, xxn
Relationships, 111
in AIDS unit, 227–231
role in, unmasking of, 204
Religiosity, 135, 138
childlike, 137
Remien, R., 69, *79*
Research, 8
Resistance, 71, 148
Restlessness, 180
Reversals, doctor–patient, 222
Ribaviran, 9
Rinaldo, C., 10, *61*
Risk, for HIV infection
acceptable level of, 50
assessing of, unconscious factors in, 46–47
exposing oneself to, 193
reduction, approach to, polarities of, 50
Risk groups for HIV, 6
Risk-taking, 49, 50, 199
romantic idealization and, 49, 50
self-delusion related to, 200
Ritalin, 134
Rituals, ceremonial, loss of, 211
Roberts, J., 91, *94*
Role
dependent, change of, 104
exploration of, 198
reversal, 75
Role relationships, 234
in AIDS unit, 229
Romantic idealization, risk-taking and, 49, 50
Rotello, G., 51, *61*
Rowland, C., 28, *61*
Ruprecht, R., 51, *58*
Rutan, J. S., 183, 186, *190*
Rutherford, G., 51, *60*
Ryan, S., 82, 93, *94*

S

Saakvitne, K., 172, *174*
Sad feelings, dissociation from, 159
Sadness, 78
Safe, safer sex, 71, 210
barriers to, 49
education on, 9, 103
negotiating for, 48–52
Safrit, J., 12n, *58*
Saliva exercises, 151
Samuel, M., 51, *61*
San Francisco City Clinic cohort study, 12n, 13n
Sandler, J., 218, *220*
Santorelli, M., 189, *191*
Sapphire, 84, *95*
Sarcoma, *See* Kaposi's sarcoma
Scalise, P., 48, *59*
Schaffner, B., xvii, *xxv*, 19, *61*, 209, *220*
Schrager, L., 12n, *61*
Schwartzberg, S., 22, *61*
Scott, G., 48, *58*
Sechehaye, M., 26. *62*
Secrecy, 88
Self
all-me, 106
bad, 104, 111
bad-me, 106
good-me, 106

Self *(continued)*
internalized, critical, 155
not-me, 106
return to, 100
sense of
balanced, 104
development of, 86
maintenance of, 85
recapturing and restoring of, 206
undermining of, 197
sexual, suppression of, 153
use of, in creating effective working alliance, 101–102
Self-assertiveness, difficulties in, 195
Self-blame, 185n
Self-consciousness, 196
Self-deprecating feelings, 104
Self-destructive behavior
addressing of, in sexually-compulsive gay man, 149
incorporation of AIDS into, 47
Self-direction, patient's, restoring of, 68–69
Self-display, need for, 181, 181n, 182n
Self-esteem, deficient, 156
Self-experience, 103
Self-expression, 106
Self-fulfillment, 131
Self-hatred, 101
Self-image, improvement of, 70
Self-other differentiation, 86
Self-recrimination, seroconversion during psychotherapy and, 202
Self-regulation issues, sexual compulsivity and, 156
Self-revelation, 64–65
Senterfitt, W., 51, *62*
Seroconversion
timing for, 41
Session, transcriptions of, 66
Sex
anonymous, 151
after session, 149
melding intimacy to, 155
talk of, 159
in treatment of sexually compulsive HIV-positive gay man, 153–154
Sex acts, safety of, 121
Sexual abuse, history of, in sexually compulsive HIV-positive gay man, 144, 148
Sexual affair, extramarital, 128, 129
Sexual behavior
of HIV-positive patient, exploring of, therapist's avoidance of, 74
nonrisky, 50
therapist's moral judgments on, 148
Sexual freedom, 55
Sexual identity
feminine, 230
heterosexual leader's revealing of, 214
learned versus innate, 214–216
Sexual orientation, group leader's countertransference and, 188
Sexual pattern, changes in, 75
Sexual practices, questions about, 71
Sexual preference, struggle with, 98
Sexually abused patients, shame in, 158
Sexually compulsive HIV-positive gay man, transference-countertransference configuration in treatment of, case study, 143, 160–161
history, 144–146
treatment
dissociation through drug abuse and acting out, 158–159
issue of humanness in, 146–148
sexual compulsivity and aggression, 148–156
sexual compulsivity and

self-regulation issues, 156
shame, 157–158
Sexually ritualized sequence, in compulsive behavior, 156
Sexually transmitted diseases (STDs), 55, 117, *See also* specific disease
AIDS as, 52
in future, 55
limiting future epidemics of, 56
Shame
relieving of, 69–70
in sexually compulsive gay man, 157–158
source of, 70
Shattered meaning, 22
Shenon, P., 5, *62*
Shernoff, M., 33, *62*
Shiboski, S., 51, *61*
Shilts, R., 8, *62*
Sifneos, P.E., 212, *220*
Significant other, avoiding of HIV-positive patient, 99
Significant other-pairing, 103
Silence, anger expressed through, 229
Sim, M., 48, *59*
Sleek, S., 183, *191*
Sloase, M., 48, *59*
Socarides, C., 215, *220*
Social agencies, patient's meshing with, 168
Social change, need for, 55–56
Social encounter, questions related to, 210
Social issues, applying psychoanalytic thinking to, xx
Social status, descent in, 196
Socioeconomic status, fear of AIDS and, 48
Sontag, S., 53, *62*, 188, *191*
South Africans, fear of AIDS in, 48
Speed, T., 51, *61*
Sperling, R., 48, *58*
Spiegel, D., 24, *62*, 184, *191*
Spirituality group, 103
Spitz, R., 82, *95*
Spouse, of HIV-negative person, risk-taking behavior by, 194
Status, loss of, 210–212
Sterba, R. F., 184n, *191*
Stern, D., xxiv, *xxv*
Stiehm, E., 48, 59
Stigma, 64
Stolorow, R. D., 181n, *191*
view on self-display, 181n, 182n
Straight, coming out as, 213
Strength, waning, 171
Strengths and weaknesses, integration of, 104–105
Stress, 64
Substance abuse, 185, 206
Substance abusers, HIV-positive, *See also* Intravenous drug abusers
dissociation through, 158–159
interpersonal therapeutic approach to, 98–99. 110–112
adaptations of psychotherapy, *See also* Individual psychotherapy
adaptations to psychotherapy, 105–110
creating an alliance, 99–105, *See also* Therapeutic alliance
patient population, 97–98
Successes, 131
Suicidal behavior, integration of AIDS risk into, 47
Suicidal ideation, 37–38
Suicidal thoughts, 225
Suicide, preparation for, 38
Sullivan, H. S., xx, xxiv, *xxv*, 13, *62*, 98, 102, 106, *112*
concept of person's inherent will to health, 71
definition of chumship, 102,102n
fighting of prejudice by, xxn
homosexuality of, xx
notion of not-me, 4, 5
Supervision
for heterosexual leader of gay

Supervision *(continued)*
men's bereavement group, 213
therapist's own fear of AIDS, 42, 43
Support
breaches in, in children of parents with AIDS, 86
in group process, 178
need for, 138
patient's seeking of, 24
seeking psychotherapy for, 23
Support groups, 15
Body Positive 12-week, 205
for children of parents with AIDS, 92
dynamically oriented, 206
Support network, independent, 27
Support system
interpersonal, 176
reliable, need for, 180
Supportive psychotherapy, technique for, 24
Suramin, 9
Survival time, effect of psychological treatment on, 24–25
Survivors, repeated, 31–36
Symbolization, 151–152
Symptom
in parents, effect on attachment, 90
treating of, 226
worsening, rage related to, 186–187
Symptomatology, xxiii
Syphilis, 55
AIDS and, 52–54
stages of, 52
Syphilis spirochete, 53, 54
Szalita, A., *62*, 83, 86, *95*

T

T-cell count, 11, 126, 167
effect of pregnancy on, 129
Taboo, inner, 69
Taboo behaviors, exposure to, 100
Talking, need for, in HIV patient, 65
Teenagers, *See* Adolescent
Tension regulation, deficient, 156
Termination date, arbitrary, setting of, 18
Testing procedures, 45, *See also* HIV antibody testing
Therapeutic alliance, creating of, in HIV-positive substance abusers, 99–101
creating chumship, 102–103
creating reality issues, 103–104
integration, 104–105
use of self in, 101–102
Therapeutic relationship, in managing chronic loss and grief, 171–172
Therapist
as advisor, 68
anger toward, 155
beliefs and feelings concerning death and dying, 76–79
concurrent, working with, 22
contrapuntal needs in, 173–174, *See also* Chronic loss and grief
differences for treating AIDS patient, 64
expression of emotions, 101–102
fear of contagion, 19, 42
fear of death, dealing with, 28
as helping other, 152
"heterosexism," 212
HIV test for, 42
involvement with people in patient's life, 135
knowledge required for, 13
love inherent in being, 227
as moral policeman, 74–75
patient's basic questions about, 138
patient's nickname for, 102
perceived role of, in patient becoming HIV-positive during psychotherapy, 199–200

personal losses, reliving of, 173
powerlessness of, 75
prejudices and misconceptions of, 118
questions of, *See also* Probing
HIV patient experience of, 70
relationship to disease and health, 41
relationship with, xxiii
responses, patient's control of, 147
role of, 26–27
new and unaccustomed, 65
unaccustomed, 72–73
self-revelation by, *See* Self-revelation
sense of risk of HIV infection, 41–42
sharing public shame about AIDS, xix
special listening by, 66
splitting in, 34–36
survivor guilt in, 34
task of, 27–28
as teacher, 68
therapeutically neutral position of, 26
touching and hugging by, 67–68
working with AIDS patient, chronic loss faced by, 164, *See also* Chronic loss and grief
workload of, adding to, 73
Therapist-patient relationship, 234
Therapy, *See* Psychotherapy
Thermal treatment of blood, 9
Thinking, 4
irrational, aroused by AIDS, 4
positive, 10, 10n
Thoughts, therapist's, 14
"Threshold people," 99, *See also* Liminality
Time frame, for treatment of HIV-positive patient, 64
Time-pressure psychoanalysis, 18
Todd, J., 10, *61*
Touching, patient's request for, 67, 68
Training programs, for bereavement groups, 212
Transdermal patches, 125, 126
Transference
analysis of, xxiii
mourning and, 84
complementary to, 16
effect of touching on, 67
in sexually compulsive gay man, 157
Transference reactions, 14
Transference-countertransference, *See also under* Sexually compulsive HIV-positive gay man
enactment, object constancy development through, 154, 156
Traumatization, vicarious, description of, 172–173
Treatment, *See also* specific type of treatment
failures in, historical perspective, 9–10
outcomes of, 131
refusal of, 226
Treatment issues, expectable, in HIV-positive patient, 120
Treatment team, therapist as part of, 72, 73
Treponema pallidum, 53
Tuberculosis, 97
Tucker, E., 48, *59*
Tunnell, G., 178, 179, 186, *191*
Turner, V., 99, *112*
12-step meetings, 206
Twinship, gay friendship as, 229, 229n

U

Uncertainty, toleration of, 69–70, 225
Uniqueness, 197
U.S. Congress, discouragement of AIDS prevention programs by, 8–9
Universality, 232

Unsafe sex, practice of, 38–39

V

Vaccarezza, M., 12n, *61*
Vaginal intercourse, heterosexual, unprotected, chance of HIV transmission by, 40
Van Dyke, R., 48, *58*
Veterans Administration, treatment at, 168
Victim, patient as, 197
Villinger, F., 13n, 14, *58*
Vinogradov, S., 212, *220*
Viral load, markers for, 10
Vocabulary, patient's, therapist's use of, 71
Volkan, V., 215, *220*
Vulnerability, 230
Vygotsky, L.S., 229, *235*

W

Walker, G., 19, *62*
Warmth, need for, 71
Warne, P., 50, *59*
Washington, R. A., 5, 50, *62*
Weed, S., 123
Weiler, P., 42, *61*
Western countries, AIDS in, 12
White, R., 10, *61*
Whiting, R., 91, *94*
Will, gay men dying without, 30
William Alanson White Institute, xix
  HIV Clinical Service of, xix, xx, 167, 210
Wilson, C., 69, *79*
Winiarski, M. G., 182, 189, *191*
Winkellstein, W., 51, *61*
Wish-fulfillment attitude, related to HIV infection, 4
Withdrawal
  anger expressed through, 229
  complementary, 16
Wolfenstein, M., 83, 84, 86, 87, *95*
Women
  with AIDS
    contracting of disease, 185n
    historical perspective, 6
    loneliness of, 25
    marriage for, 122–123
    misdiagnosis of, 52–53
  HIV infection in
    false beliefs related to, 7
    pregnancy in, 48
    prenancy in, 129
    transmission to child, 48
  incidence of AIDS in, 82
  unprotected vaginal intercourse in, chance of HIV infection by, 40
Word games, 106
Work, meaningful, 131
"Worried well," 5–6, 211, 211n
Worth, sense of, restoring of, 66
Worthlessness feelings, 108
Wyand, M., 51, *58*
Wypijewska, C., 40, *58*

Y

Yalom, I. D., 92, *95*, 184, *191*, 212, *220*
Yamamoto, J., 31, *62*
Yingling, S., 50, *59*
Yoshimura, S., 31, *62*
Young people, HIV infection in, 6

Z

Zhang, L., 12n, *58*